Fast Facts

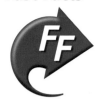

D0785698

Fast Facts:
Urology Highlights
2005–06

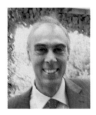

Edited by Julian Shah FRCS

Senior Lecturer and Honorary Consultant Urologist
Institute of Urology and Nephrology
University College London, UK

HEALTH PRESS

Fast Facts: Urology Highlights 2005–06
First published March 2006

© 2006 in this edition Health Press Limited
Health Press Limited, Elizabeth House, Queen Street, Abingdon,
Oxford OX14 3LN, UK
Tel: +44 (0)1235 523233
Fax: +44 (0)1235 523238

Book orders can be placed by telephone or via the website.
For regional distributors or to order via the website, please go to:
www.fastfacts.com
For telephone orders, please call 01752 202301 (UK), +44 1752 202301 (Europe),
1 800 247 6553 (USA, toll free) or +1 419 281 1802 (Americas).

Fast Facts is a trademark of Health Press Limited.

A CIP record for this title is available from the British Library.

ISBN 1-903734-84-3

Shah, J (Julian)
Fast Facts: Urology Highlights 2005–06/
Julian Shah

Typesetting and page layout by Zed, Oxford, UK.
Printed by Fine Print (Services) Ltd, Oxford, UK.

Printed with vegetable inks on fully biodegradable and
recyclable paper manufactured from sustainable forests.

444   001

Low emissions
during production

Low
chlorine

Sustainable
forests

Introduction

This year's edition of *Fast Facts: Urology Highlights* is the tenth – an exciting milestone. The idea of an annual review of the highlights in our field was spawned from the fact that we learn much from meetings but many papers never see the light of day. A great deal of very useful and topical information is thus 'lost' every year. Abstracts from meetings are not usually read after the event and are not quoted as part of the literature. Hence the *Urology Highlights* series brings you up-to-date research from the major meetings each year, selected by a panel of international experts who work hard to bring this information to you with a tight deadline. It is rare to find people who can turn around a chapter from request to print in 2 or 3 months, and I am grateful to them all.

I hope you find this year's edition of *Urology Highlights* useful in extending your understanding of our exciting specialty of urology, and that you will continue to support the venture.

Julian Shah FRCS
Institute of Urology and Nephrology
University College London, UK

Basic science

Paul Cathcart MBBS MRCS, James Armitage MBBS MRCS and
Mark Emberton MD FRCS(Urol)
Institute of Urology and Nephrology, London, UK

There have been many advances in the basic science of urology
over the last year. This chapter focuses on published research with
potential clinical applications.

Bladder physiology

Management of the overactive bladder requires an understanding
of the neurophysiological mechanisms involved in normal function
of the bladder. These processes are complex and remain poorly
understood. The mainstay of pharmacological therapy involves
the use of antimuscarinic agents. The muscarinic M_3 receptor
subtype mediates detrusor smooth-muscle contraction; thus efforts
have been directed at targeting this receptor selectively in order
to reduce the adverse events of systemic antimuscarinic agents.
Recent studies have shown that the selective M_3 receptor
antagonists darifenacin and solifenacin are safe and effective
and that their adverse-event profiles are better than those of
non-selective antimuscarinic agents.[1,2]

The possible role of the M_2 receptor subtype has also attracted
attention. A high density of M_2 receptors has been identified in
human bladder detrusor smooth muscle and mucosa.[3] Possible
mechanisms of action of this receptor include enhancement of the
M_3-receptor-mediated contraction[4] and inhibition of the adenosine-
receptor- and beta-adrenoceptor-evoked relaxation[5] of the detrusor
muscle.

There is continued interest in the use of botulinum toxin for
patients with symptoms that are refractory to first-line medication.[6]
Intrinsic pacemaker cells within the detrusor muscle have been
identified, similar to the interstitial cells of Cajal found in the bowel

wall, and might direct future therapy.[7] Research into the role of the central nervous system and urothelial-derived mediators in the overactive bladder continues.

Urinary tract infections

Antibiotic resistance in pathogenic organisms that cause recurrent urinary tract infections (UTIs) is a growing problem for the urologist. It has led to the development of a number of non-antimicrobial therapies. Several studies have investigated the possibility of developing vaccines[8,9] to protect against the common uropathogens such as *Escherichia coli*. These vaccines are likely to be based on adhesion molecules such as FimH adhesin that mediate the binding of *E. coli* fimbriae (type 1) to uroplakin, found in the uroepithelium of the bladder. The sequencing of FimH has allowed antiserum to be raised, which in turn has been shown to inhibit adherence of *E. coli*.[10] Vaccines based on adhesins such as FimH therefore represent a potential method for preventing UTI.

Another example of a non-antimicrobial therapy to combat UTI, this time in the catheterized patient, is iontophoresis. This involves passing an electric current through silver electrodes attached to a catheter (the 'electrified catheter'). In a recent study, iontophoresis was found to reduce urinary bacterial colony counts and to prevent bacterial encrustation of urinary catheters by releasing ions into the urine.[11]

Oncology

There have been considerable advances in the molecular diagnosis and staging of urologic cancer. Several studies have evaluated the use of various molecular markers in attempts to improve detection of bladder cancer and to stratify patients into high and low risk for tumor recurrence/progression.

In a recent study of 209 cases, the presence of survivin, a protein that regulates cell death by inhibiting apoptosis, was found to be a stronger independent predictor of the presence of bladder cancer than was urine cytology, having a sensitivity of 64% and a specificity of 93%.[12] Furthermore, higher urinary levels of survivin were associated with higher grade of disease, although levels of survivin were not found to rise with increasing stage of disease.

Another promising novel molecular marker is the BLCA-1 protein. This protein, detected in the urine using an immunoblot assay generated from antibodies produced by BLCA-1 sequence data, has recently been shown to have a high sensitivity (80%) and specificity (87%) for detection of bladder cancer.[13]

A further non-invasive molecular test is fluorescence in situ hybridization (FISH). This test, designed to detect aneusomy of chromosomes 3, 7 and 17, as well as the loss of the 9p21 locus, has recently been shown to aid categorization of patients into high and low risk for disease progression/recurrence, according to the presence or absence of these chromosomal abnormalities in exfoliated tumor cells in voided urine.[14]

Molecular markers are also being evaluated for the detection of prostate cancer and prediction of outcome. A novel urine test designed to detect the presence of the protein α-methylacyl coenzyme A racemase (AMACR) has recently been evaluated in two studies and, when checked against prostate biopsy, had a sensitivity of 100% and a specificity of 58%.[15,16] This suggests that a screening test based on urinary AMACR may be a useful adjunct to serum prostate-specific antigen testing for identifying men who are at an increased risk of harboring cancer despite a negative biopsy.

Molecular markers for monitoring outcomes after therapy have also recently been reported. Using tissue microarray analysis, the expression of *hMSH2*, an example of a mismatch repair gene, has been shown to differ in malignant prostate tissue. The staining intensity of *hMSH2* correlated with Gleason score as well as with overall and disease-free survival.[17] Furthermore, the degree of *hMSH2* expression has been found to correlate with time to biochemical recurrence following prostatectomy.

Future molecular research is likely to include microarray transcript expression profiling, which is able to profile, qualitatively and quantitatively, genes expressed within different malignant tissues of the urinary tract.

Highlights in **basic science** 2005–06

WHAT'S IN?

- M_3 and M_2 receptor blockade within the bladder for detrusor instability
- Molecular markers for the diagnosis and staging of urologic malignancy

WHAT'S ON THE HORIZON?

- Microarray-based transcript expression profiling of genes expressed within malignant tissues

Erectile dysfunction

Physical organic causes are thought to account for the majority of cases of erectile dysfunction, although psychological components often contribute.[18] Normal erectile function requires the synthesis of nitric oxide (NO) from L-arginine, with the subsequent accumulation of cyclic guanosine monophosphate (cGMP), which mediates smooth-muscle relaxation. An understanding of the pivotal role of NO synthesis and breakdown of cGMP by phosphodiesterase-5 (PDE5) has directed therapy for erectile dysfunction. A breakthrough in the management of erectile dysfunction occurred with the introduction of the PDE5 inhibitor sildenafil nearly a decade ago. Sildenafil is effective in the majority of men with erectile dysfunction, although those with diabetic or post-prostatectomy erectile dysfunction often respond less well. The debate as to whether men develop resistance during long-term treatment with sildenafil appears to have been answered by Musicki and colleagues.[19] Using an animal model, they demonstrated that there was no tachyphylaxis with sildenafil and possibly a more pronounced effect in animals with erectile impairment than those with normal erectile ability.

Newer PDE5 inhibitors include vardenafil and tadalafil. Vardenafil has been shown to have better potency,[20] and tadalafil a longer half-life,[21] than sildenafil. However, to date all PDE5 inhibitors have been associated with adverse events such as headache, flushing, dyspepsia and nasal congestion or rhinitis, and therefore the search continues for a highly selective PDE5 inhibitor that has a more favorable adverse-event profile.[22]

NO donor drugs provide another treatment modality for the management of erectile dysfunction.[23] In rabbits with hypercholesterolemia-induced erectile dysfunction, sildenafil has been shown to have increased effectiveness in the presence of an NO donor, which may lead to the development of more effective treatments.[24]

Gene therapy is an attractive therapeutic option for erectile dysfunction. NO synthase, the enzyme that controls NO synthesis, has been the focus of many gene therapies designed to modulate erectile response. Recently a small interfering RNA (siRNA) was found to effectively downregulate PDE5 expression and so prolong cGMP expression in a rat model.[25]

References

1. Brunton S, Kuritzky L. Recent developments in the management of overactive bladder: focus on the efficacy and tolerability of once daily solifenacin succinate 5 mg. *Curr Med Res Opin* 2005;21:71–80.

2. Chapple C, Steers W, Norton P et al. A pooled analysis of three phase III studies to investigate the efficacy, tolerability and safety of darifenacin, a muscarinic M_3 selective receptor antagonist, in the treatment of overactive bladder. *BJU Int* 2005; 95:993–1001.

3. Mansfield KJ, Liu L, Mitchelson FJ, Moore KH et al. Muscarinic receptor subtypes in human bladder detrusor and mucosa, studied by radioligand binding and quantitative competitive RT-PCR: changes in ageing. *Br J Pharmacol* 2005;144:1089–99.

4. Ehlert FJ, Griffin MT, Abe DM et al. The M_2 muscarinic receptor mediates contraction through indirect mechanisms in mouse urinary bladder. *J Pharmacol Exp Ther* 2005;313:368–78.

5. Giglio D, Delbro DS, Tobin G. Postjunctional modulation by muscarinic M_2 receptors of responses to electrical field stimulation of rat detrusor muscle preparations. *Auton Autacoid Pharmacol* 2005;25: 113–20.

6. Ghei M, Maraj BH, Miller R et al. Effects of botulinum toxin B on refractory detrusor overactivity: a randomized, double-blind, placebo controlled, crossover trial. *J Urol* 2005;174:1873–7.

7. Biers S, Reynard J, Doore T, Brading A. Inhibition of spontaneous activity and contractility in guinea-pig and human detrusor using a c-kit receptor blocker. *XXth Congress of the European Association of Urology* 2005;4:70.

8. Li X, Erbe JL, Lockatell CV, Johnson DE et al. Use of translational fusion of the MrpH fimbrial adhesin-binding domain with the cholera toxin A2 domain, coexpressed with the cholera toxin B subunit, as an intranasal vaccine to prevent experimental urinary tract infection by *Proteus mirabilis*. *Infect Immun* 2004;72:7306–10.

9. Langermann S, Ballou WR. Development of a recombinant FimCH vaccine for urinary tract infections. *Adv Exp Med Biol* 2003;539(Pt B):635–48.

10. Meiland R, Geerlings SE, Langermann S et al. FimCH antiserum inhibits the adherence of *Escherichia coli* to cells collected by voided urine specimens of diabetic women. *J Urol* 2004;171:1589–93.

11. Chakravarti A, Gangodawila S, Long MJ et al. An electrified catheter to resist encrustation by *Proteus mirabilis* biofilm. *J Urol* 2005;174: 1129–32.

12. Shariat SF, Casella R, Khoddami SM et al. Urine detection of survivin is a sensitive marker for the noninvasive diagnosis of bladder cancer. *J Urol* 2004;171:626–30.

13. Myers-Irvin JM, Landsittel D, Getzenberg RH. Use of the novel marker BLCA-1 for the detection of bladder cancer. *J Urol* 2005;174: 64–8.

14. Bollmann M, Heller H, Bankfalvi A et al. Quantitative molecular urinary cytology by fluorescence in situ hybridization: a tool for tailoring surveillance of patients with superficial bladder cancer? *BJU Int* 2005;95:1219–25.

15. Rogers CG, Yan G, Zha S et al. Prostate cancer detection on urinalysis for α methylacyl coenzyme A racemase protein. *J Urol* 2004; 172:1501–3.

16. Zielie PJ, Mobley JA, Ebb RG et al. A novel diagnostic test for prostate cancer emerges from the determination of alpha-methylacyl-coenzyme A racemase in prostatic secretions. *J Urol* 2004;172:1130–3.

17. Prtilo A, Leach FS, Markwalder R et al. Tissue microarray analysis of *hMSH2* expression predicts outcome in men with prostate cancer. *J Urol* 2005;174:1814–18; discussion 1818.

18. Wyllie MG. The underlying pathophysiology and causes of erectile dysfunction. *Clin Cornerstone* 2005;7:19–27.

19. Musicki B, Champion HC, Becker RE et al. In vivo analysis of chronic phosphodiesterase-5 inhibition with sildenafil in penile erectile tissues: no tachyphylaxis effect. *J Urol* 2005;174:1493–6.

20. Corbin JD, Beasley A, Blount MA, Francis SH. Vardenafil: structural basis for higher potency over sildenafil in inhibiting cGMP-specific phosphodiesterase-5 (PDE5). *Neurochem Int* 2004;45:859–63.

21. Young JM, Feldman RA, Auerbach SM et al. Tadalafil improved erectile function at twenty-four and thirty-six hours after dosing in men with erectile dysfunction: US trial. *J Androl* 2005;26:310–18.

22. Boyle CD, Xu R, Asberom T et al. Optimization of purine based PDE1/PDE5 inhibitors to a potent and selective PDE5 inhibitor for the treatment of male ED. *Bioorg Med Chem Lett* 2005;15:2365–9.

23. Scatena R, Bottoni P, Martorana GE, Giardina B. Nitric oxide donor drugs: an update on pathophysiology and therapeutic potential. *Expert Opin Invest Drugs* 2005;14:835–46.

24. Shukla N, Jones R, Persad R et al. Effect of sildenafil citrate and a nitric oxide donating sildenafil derivative, NCX 911, on cavernosal relaxation and superoxide formation in hypercholesterolaemic rabbits. *Eur J Pharmacol* 2005;517:224–31.

25. Lin G, Hayashi N, Carrion R et al. Improving erectile function by silencing phosphodiesterase-5. *J Urol* 2005;174:1142–8.

Navroop Johal MRCS, Divyesh Desai FRCS and Peter Cuckow FRCS

Department of Paediatric Urology, Great Ormond Street Hospital, London, UK

Posterior urethral valves

Posterior urethral valve (PUV) is the most common cause of lower urinary obstruction resulting in end-stage renal failure.[1] The prognosis for these patients has improved dramatically over the last half-century because of improvements in diagnosis through prenatal screening, advances in surgical techniques for valve ablation and a better understanding of the pathophysiology of the disease process.

Prognostic markers. End-stage renal damage occurs in up to 33% of patients with PUV.[1] A number of prognostic markers are used in the monitoring of such patients, including grade of vesicoureteric reflux (VUR), reduction in glomerular filtration rate (GFR), renal scarring and rises in serum creatinine concentration. Bajpai and colleagues have recently suggested that these markers enable detection of renal damage only when the disease is severe, and have proposed plasma renin activity (PRA) as a useful marker. They studied PRA in a series of 14 patients with renal damage and found it to be raised in all nine of the patients who had normal GFR.[2] A long-term review of 54 boys with PUV emphasized the importance of regular assessment of renal and bladder function to improve the long-term prognosis.[3]

Surgery. Valve ablation is the treatment of choice in patients with PUV. Ghanem and Nijman examined the effect of bilateral high ureterostomies in 36 patients and found that it immediately releases high intrarenal pressures. However, it improves renal function in the short term only and may merely temporarily delay the onset of end-stage renal disease.[4]

Hypospadias

Hypospadias occurs in nearly 1 in 250 live births and has a wide range of severity.[5] The goal of any treatment is a penis with normal appearance and function. Most hypospadiac deformities can be corrected successfully in a single-stage procedure, but lately there has been much debate over the correction of the more severe proximal forms.

Single-stage or two-stage repair? Recently, there have been reports of successful single-stage repairs of severe proximal hypospadias using the tubularized preputial island flaps.[6] Patel and colleagues reported success using the vascularized flap in a series of 12 patients. Although these results are encouraging, other series using similar flap techniques have reported complication rates of 33–90%.[7,8] Nuininga and colleagues looked at the long-term results of all single-stage procedures in 2000 patients and concluded that, even in the hands of experienced pediatric urologists, the complication rate following repair remains high, with an average of 54% at 10-year follow-up.[9]

The two-stage repair has been said to provide far superior cosmetic and functional results than does the single-stage procedure using onlay flaps.[10] Johal et al. reviewed a cohort of 62 patients who underwent two-stage reconstruction for severe primary hypospadias and concluded it is a reliable, reproducible technique with a low complication rate.[11] Similarly, Lam and colleagues looked at the long-term results (mean follow-up of 12.7 years) of the two-stage technique for the repair of severe proximal hypospadias in 44 patients and concluded that it offers excellent function, cosmesis and patient satisfaction after puberty.[12]

Antibiotic prophylaxis. A prospective study comparing postoperative prophylactic antibiotics with no antibiotics concluded that the former may reduce the risk of urinary tract infection after surgery, and probably reduces meatal stenosis and urethrocutaneous fistula rates.[13]

Exstrophy–epispadias complex

Management of bladder exstrophy (BE) presents several challenges, beginning with initial repair using the conventional staged approach or the recently described complete primary repair technique.

Complete primary repair of bladder exstrophy (CPRE) is a relatively new approach in the long history of BE treatment. CPRE includes repair of the epispadias component of the defect at initial surgery, funneling the bladder neck and, in some cases, reimplanting the ureters.[14] Borer and colleagues looked at 23 newborns with BE who underwent CPRE. With the number of additional early procedures required, such as hypospadias repair and ureteral reimplantation, the authors recommended reimplantation at the time of closure to protect the upper tracts and reduce the need for an additional procedure. They concluded that, over the 8-year period, complication rates were similar to those associated with the staged approach. Continence can be achieved with additional surgical procedures, such as bladder-neck reconstruction. The same authors have shown that the staged approach provides a larger bladder capacity than does CPRE, but detrusor overactivity was reduced in the CPRE group.[15]

New surgical techniques for the management of BE are being developed. Mathews and Gearhart have stated that the standard these 'newer' techniques need to reach remains that of the modern staged reconstruction,[16] although as more experience is gained with these procedures, they may eventually replace the current gold standard of staged reconstruction.

The Kelly repair. Following neonatal primary closure, the Kelly repair provides radical soft-tissue reconstruction of BE without involving osteotomies. After the bladder is opened and the ureters reimplanted, the urethral plate is separated from the penile shaft skin and lifted off the corpora to the level of the bladder neck. Following bladder closure, the perineal muscle is wrapped around the urethra below the corpora.[17] The Kelly repair has been shown to create a reliable, controllable outlet resistance in an unselected cohort of 23 children.[18]

Long-term outcomes. Baird and colleagues have looked at long-term outcomes in a group of patients with BE treated between 1960 and 1982. The patients are healthy and well-adjusted individuals, functioning well in society, often in full-time employment and long-term relationships.[19] The same authors also reviewed 25 patients who remained incontinent into adolescence, all of whom achieved continence through modern reconstructive techniques.[20]

Vesicoureteral reflux

The consequences of untreated VUR include urinary tract infection, hypertension, renal scarring and reflux nephropathy.

Prenatal diagnosis. Penido Silva and colleagues evaluated the clinical course of prenatally detected primary VUR over an 8-year period.[21] Fifty-three children (41 boys) with VUR detected by investigation of prenatal hydronephrosis were followed up for a mean time of 66 months. During the follow-up, the clinical outcome of the VUR was relatively benign. Renal function remained within normal limits in all patients and no new renal scars developed. However, despite prophylactic antibiotics from the first day of life in most patients, 25% of children had breakthrough urinary tract infections during follow-up.[21]

Imaging in familial VUR. The incidence of VUR in siblings of children with VUR is 26–51%.[22] Giel and colleagues have examined the outcomes of a conventional ultrasound screening program in older asymptomatic siblings. Eleven out of a total of 117 siblings were referred for a voiding cystourethrogram (VCUG). The authors concluded that observation alone is an acceptable form of management in this group, given the innocuous nature of VUR in older asymptomatic siblings of known patients with reflux. However, if there is either parental or physician anxiety about this approach, conventional ultrasonography offers a reliable alternative to invasive VCUG screening.[22]

Treatment. Correction of VUR through endoscopic injection into the subureteric space has become an established alternative to long-term antibiotic prophylaxis and open surgical treatment. Keating suggested that medical management is favored when the chances of spontaneous resolution are high and the anticipated length of therapy is short.[23] When medical management is not an option, open surgery provides the most effective solution. Injection therapy offers a less effective solution for reflux.[23]

Stones

Management of pediatric urolithiasis has evolved from open surgery to minimally invasive techniques such as extracorporeal shock-wave lithotripsy (ESWL). In children, clinical manifestations of stone disease are often more subtle than the dramatic adult presentation.[24]

Raza and colleagues looked at 122 children with calculi varying in size from 6 to 110 mm over a 15-year period.[25] For the majority of renal stones smaller than 20 mm, ESWL was the most effective primary treatment modality. For stones 20 mm or greater and staghorn calculi, percutaneous nephrostolithotomy (PCNL) was the preferred treatment modality. Holmium laser lithotripsy was a primary treatment modality for ureteral stones, decreasing the number of re-treatments required. Sternberg and colleagues reviewed their 12-year experience of stone management and concluded that half of the patients passed the stones and ESWL was curative in most of the other cases. Ureteroscopy, PCNL and open surgery were rarely required.[26]

Laparoscopy

The introduction of laparoscopy and robotic-assisted techniques has allowed minimally invasive reconstructive surgery that mirrors open surgical procedures. These techniques offer substantial benefits to patients by reducing morbidity, accelerating postoperative recovery, causing less pain and improving cosmetic outcome.

Highlights in **pediatric urology** 2005–06

WHAT'S IN?

- Laparoscopic retroperitoneal pyeloplasty
- Extracorporeal shock-wave lithotripsy for renal stones smaller than 20 mm

WHAT'S OUT?

- Voiding cystourethrogram as a primary screening tool for vesicoureteral reflux

WHAT'S NEW?

- Robotic-assisted surgery
- Prophylactic antibiotics following hypospadias repair
- Plasma renin activity as a prognostic marker in posterior urethral valves
- Kelly procedure for bladder exstrophy

WHAT'S CONTROVERSIAL?

- Single-stage versus two-stage repair of severe primary hypospadias
- Bilateral high ureterostomies in the treatment of posterior urethral valves
- Transperitoneal or retroperitoneal approach for laparoscopic pyeloplasty

Laparoscopic retroperitoneal pyeloplasty (LRP). Bonnard and colleagues compared 22 children undergoing LRP and 17 children undergoing open-flank pyeloplasty. The operative time was longer with LRP, but the main advantages were significantly reduced hospital stay and analgesic use compared with the open procedure.[27] The debate over transperitoneal or retroperitoneal approach continues, but the transperitoneal approach theoretically increases the risk of abdominal organ injury; it requires more dissection to reach the kidney, and the colon must be reflected. The main disadvantages of the laparoscopic approach are longer operative time and the long learning curve, making the teaching process more difficult and problematic. These disadvantages might be improved by the new robotic-assisted equipment.[27]

Robotic-assisted laparoscopic pyeloplasty. There have been numerous reports of transperitoneal laparoscopic pyeloplasty in adults and older children. However, there have been few series of robotic-assisted laparoscopic pyeloplasty in young children. Atug and colleagues reported their experience with 7 children undergoing robotic-assisted laparoscopic pyeloplasty. Mean operative time, including setting up the robot, was 184 minutes, and mean anastomosis time was 39 minutes; no additional procedures were required postoperatively.[28]

References

1. Parkhouse HF, Barratt TM, Dillon MJ et al. Long-term outcome of boys with posterior urethral valves. *BJU* 1988;621:59–62.

2. Bajpai M, Pratap A, Tripathi M, Bal CS. Posterior urethral valves: preliminary observations on the significance of plasma renin activity as a prognostic marker. *J Urol* 2005;173:592–4.

3. Holmdahl G, Sillen U. Boys with posterior urethral valves: outcome concerning renal function, bladder function and paternity at ages 31 to 44 years. *J Urol* 2005;174:1031–4.

4. Ghanem MA, Nijman RJ. Long-term followup of bilateral high (sober) urinary diversion in patients with posterior urethral valves and its effect on bladder function. *J Urol* 2005;173:1721–4.

5. Duckett JW. Hypospadias. In: Walsh PC, Retik AB, Vaughan ED et al., eds. *Campbell's Urology*, 7th edn. Philadelphia: WB Saunders, 1998:2093–119.

6. Patel RP, Shukla AR, Austin JC, Canning DA. Modified tubularized transverse preputial island flap repair for severe proximal hypospadias. *BJU Int* 2005;956:901–4.

7. Demirbilek S, Kanmaz T, Aydin G, Yucesan S. Outcomes of one-stage techniques for proximal hypospadias repair. *Urology* 2001;582:267–70.

8. Castañón M, Muñoz E, Carrasco R et al. Treatment of proximal hypospadias with a tubularized island flap urethroplasty and the onlay technique: a comparative study. *J Pediatr Surg* 2000;35:1453–5.

9. Nuininga JE, De Gier RP, Verschuren R, Feitz WF. Long-term outcome of different types of 1-stage hypospadias repair. *J Urol* 2005;174: 1544–8; discussion 1548.

10. Gershbaum MD, Stock JA, Hanna MK. A case for 2-stage repair of perineoscrotal hypospadias with severe chordee. *J Urol* 2002;168: 1727–8.

11. Johal NS, Nitkunan T, O'Malley K, Cuckow PM. The Two-Stage Repair for Severe Primary Hypospadias. *Eur Urol* 2006; Jan 25 [epub ahead of print].

12. Lam PN, Greenfield SP, Williot P. 2-stage repair in infancy for severe hypospadias with chordee: long-term results after puberty. *J Urol* 2005; 174:1567–72.

13. Meir DB, Livne PM. Is prophylactic antimicrobial treatment necessary after hypospadias repair? *J Urol* 2004;171:2621–2.

14. Borer JG, Gargollo PC, Hendren WH et al. Early outcome following complete primary repair of bladder exstrophy in the newborn. *J Urol* 2005;174:1674–8.

15. Borer JG, Gargollo PC, Kinnamon DD et al. Bladder growth and development after complete primary repair of bladder exstrophy in the newborn with comparison to staged approach. *J Urol* 2005; 174:1553–7.

16. Mathews R, Gearhart JP. Modern staged reconstruction of bladder exstrophy – still the gold standard. *Urology* 2005;651:2–4.

17. Kelly J, Cuckow P, Desai D. Radical soft tissue reconstruction for continence in bladder exstrophy (Kelly's operation). *J Pediatr Urol* 2005;13:183–4.

18. Cuckow P, Desai D. Continence following soft tissue reconstruction (Kelly's operation) in unselected cases of classic bladder exstrophy. *J Pediatr Urol* 2005;13:184.

19. Baird AD, Sanders C, Woolfenden A, Gearhart JP. Coping with bladder exstrophy: diverse results from early attempts at functional urinary tract surgery. *BJU Int* 2004;939:1303–8.

20. Baird AD, Frimberger D, Gearhart JP. Reconstructive lower urinary tract surgery in incontinent adolescents with exstrophy/epispadias complex. *Urology* 2005;663:636–40.

21. Penido Silva JM, Oliveira EA, Diniz JS et al. Clinical course of prenatally detected primary vesicoureteral reflux. *Pediatr Nephrol* 2006;21:86–91.

22. Giel DW, Noe HN, Williams MA. Ultrasound screening of asymptomatic siblings of children with vesicoureteral reflux: a long-term followup study. *J Urol* 2005;174:1602–4.

23. Keating MA. Role of periureteral injections in children with vesicoureteral reflux. *Curr Opin Urol* 2005;156:369–73.

24. Bartosh SM. Medical management of pediatric stone disease. *Urol Clin North Am* 2004;31:575–87;x–xi.

25. Raza A, Turna B, Smith G et al. Pediatric urolithiasis: 15 years of local experience with minimally invasive endourological management of pediatric calculi. *J Urol* 2005;174:682–5.

26. Sternberg K, Greenfield SP, Williot P, Wan J. Pediatric stone disease: an evolving experience. *J Urol* 2005;174:1711–14.

27. Bonnard A, Fouquet V, Carricaburu E et al. Retroperitoneal laparoscopic versus open pyeloplasty in children. *J Urol* 2005;173:1710–13.

28. Atug F, Woods M, Burgess SV et al. Robotic assisted laparoscopic pyeloplasty in children. *J Urol* 2005;174:1440–2.

Neurogenic bladder

Michael J Schwartz MD, Ricardo R Gonzalez MD,
Jeffrey P Weiss MD FACS and Jerry G Blaivas MD FACS
James Buchanan Brady Department of Urology, New York Presbyterian
Hospital–Weill Cornell Medical Center, New York, NY, USA

Over the past year, great strides in the diagnosis and management of neurogenic bladder were made. Novel techniques have allowed for preliminary non-invasive urodynamic evaluation. Experience with botulinum toxin is maturing, with new basic science insights into its effects and confirmed efficacy in children with neurogenic bladders. Combination medical therapy with α-adrenergic and muscarinic antagonists is coming of age in the treatment of neurogenic voiding dysfunction. Basic science is elucidating the effects of age and hormonal milieu on neurogenic bladder dysfunction and the response to medical therapy. New classes of medications for the treatment of detrusor overactivity and bladder inflammation are surfacing. Of surgical therapies, preliminary experience with pudendal nerve stimulation is most promising.

PubMed, Ovid and MEDLINE databases were searched for peer-reviewed research articles published in 2005 with keywords 'neurogenic bladder' and 'neuropathic bladder'. Over 150 articles and abstracts from major scientific meetings were reviewed, and the following studies were selected for this chapter.

Basic science

Apostolidis et al. reported on the decreased expression of the capsaicin receptor TRPV1 in urothelium of neurogenic human bladders treated with intravesical resiniferatoxin (RTX).[1] Considering that patients with neurogenic detrusor activity (NDO) have greater expression of TRPV1 than controls, TRPV1 likely plays an important role in the pathophysiology of NDO. Similarly, a separate study by Apostolidis et al. on TRPV1 and purinergic receptor P2X3 immunoreactive sensory receptors in suburothelial nerve fibers showed decreased receptor expression following intradetrusor injections of botulinum toxin A (BTX-A) for human NDO.[2] Decreased urgency was reported at 4 weeks, with more significant decrease at 16 weeks. This clinical finding was correlated with decreased expression of P2X3 and TRPV1 sensory fibers, likewise more dramatic at 16 weeks than at 4 weeks after treatment.

Giannantoni and colleagues investigated the effect of BTX-A on visceral afferent nerve transmission by measuring bladder tissue concentration of nerve growth factor (NGF) in patients with NDO before and after detrusor injections with BTX-A. BTX-A injections induced NGF deprivation in these patients, resulting in a decrease in hyperexcitability of C-fiber afferents, and clinical reduction in uninhibited detrusor contractions.[3]

Gonzalez et al. reported the efficacy of a novel class of anti-inflammatory drug, RDP58, in modulating neuroinflammation in an established murine model of cystitis. Intravesical RDP58 abolished histological inflammation and reduced production of NGF, substance P and tumor necrosis factor α.[4]

Using spinal cord injured rats with neurogenic detrusor overactivity (NDO), Abdel-Karim et al. showed a dose- and time-dependent response to a neurokinin-2 receptor antagonist for treatment of NDO.[5] The rats' bladder capacity improved and voiding pressures decreased on post-treatment urodynamics compared with pre-treatment studies. Neurokinin-2 receptor antagonists may provide an alternative to antimuscarinics for patients with NDO.

Wuest and colleagues investigated whether age affects the contractility of the human detrusor, its responsiveness to spasmolytic and cholinergic drugs (e.g. propiverine, oxybutinin, tolterodine and atropine), and expression of selective muscarinic and purinergic receptor subtypes (M2, M3, P2X1 and P2X3). Tissues from 63 patients from 37 to 84 years old undergoing radical cystectomy were used for contractility studies. Results did not provide evidence for age-related contractile deterioration in human detrusor strips, nor did they suggest that responsiveness to anticholinergic spasmolytic drugs changed significantly with age.[6]

Ahmed et al. investigated whether estrogen deficiency affected neuroregeneration and functional recovery after rat pudendal nerve injury; it resulted in a lower leak point pressure and decreased markers of nerve regeneration compared with control groups, suggesting that estrogen may promote nerve regeneration and recovery of urethral function after pudendal nerve injury.[7]

Non-invasive urodynamics

Non-invasive measurement of bladder pressure, volume and dysfunction has generated significant interest and attention in the literature for 2005.

Griffiths et al. developed a nomogram to classify men with lower urinary tract symptoms using urine flow and non-invasive measurement of bladder pressure using controlled inflation of a penile cuff.[8] The proposed nomogram combined with the additional flow-rate criterion can classify more than two-thirds of cases without recourse to invasive pressure–flow studies (Figure 1).

Two non-invasive methods of diagnosing bladder outlet obstruction (BOO) using ultrasound are proposed by Nose et al. – intravesical prostatic protrusion and velocity–flow urodynamics.[9] In the study, 30 patients underwent conventional pressure–flow urodynamics in addition to the two non-invasive approaches, which showed good sensitivity and specificity for the diagnosis of BOO.

Medical therapy

Combined therapies for voiding dysfunction. Ruggieri et al. performed a literature review of data supporting the combined use of α-adrenergic and muscarinic antagonists for the treatment of voiding dysfunction.[10] While the generally accepted physiological action of α-adrenergic antagonists comprises relaxation of periurethral, prostatic and bladder-neck smooth muscle, there is additional evidence for effect at extraprostatic sites involved in micturition – bladder-dome smooth muscle, peripheral ganglia, spinal cord and brain. Similarly, while the most well-known

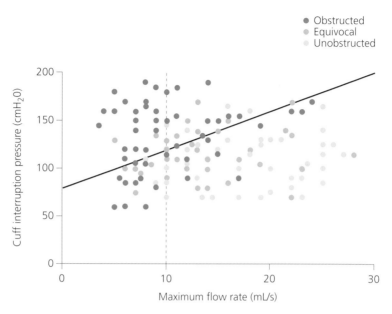

Figure 1 Pressure–flow nomogram developed by Griffiths et al.,[8] based on the International Continence Society nomogram, with data from 144 men with lower urinary tract symptoms tested in pressure–flow studies, showing its use for classifying obstruction. Reproduced with permission from the American Urological Association.

mechanism of antimuscarinics is their effect on M_3 muscarinic receptors, there is evidence that M_2 receptors, which are also affected by antimuscarinics, mediate both hypertrophied bladder contractions and supraspinal control of voiding. On this evidence, it is likely that combined therapy would be more beneficial than either alone, as they would affect two components of detrusor function.

Anticholinergics. Ellsworth and colleagues reported the relationship between the dose of tolterodine and urodynamic response in children with NDO from three separate prospective studies.[11] Studies 1 and 2, in children up to the age of 10 years and using immediate-release (IR) tolterodine, showed some dose-related increases in volume to first detrusor contraction and bladder capacity. Study 3, in children aged 11–15 years and using extended-release (ER) tolterodine, showed no dose-response urodynamic relationships. There were no adverse events in any of the studies.

Franco et al. confirmed the safety and efficacy of oxybutynin in children with detrusor hyperreflexia secondary to neurogenic bladder dysfunction.[12]

A randomized, double-blind, placebo-controlled study of darifenacin versus oxybutinin was performed on 76 patients with overactive bladder (OAB) by Zinner and colleagues.[13] Both drugs significantly reduced incontinence episodes as well as the number and severity of urgency episodes. The authors concluded that darifenacin provides equal efficacy to and greater tolerability than oxybutinin.

Kelleher et al. assessed the quality of life (QoL) in patients with OAB treated with solifenacin versus placebo in two randomized, double-blinded, multicenter trials of 1984 patients.[14] Results showed a significant improvement in QoL score in patients receiving solifenacin compared with placebo after 12 weeks and further improvement with long-term administration up to 1 year. Additionally, the authors reported a promising balance between efficacy and tolerability on the basis of improved QoL scores after both short-term and long-term administration.

Botulinum toxin. Botulinum toxin remained at the forefront in the neurogenic bladder literature in 2005. Schurch et al. published results of a randomized, placebo-controlled study of botulinum toxin type A for treatment of neurogenic urinary incontinence due to detrusor overactivity in 59 patients.[15] There were significant decreases in post-treatment incontinence episodes from baseline in the botulinum toxin group versus placebo. Benefit was observed from the first 2 weeks after treatment until the conclusion of the study at 24 weeks; results were assessed both by QoL questionnaires and urodynamic evaluation showing improved bladder function. In a subanalysis presented at the American Urological Association annual meeting, sex and age were reported not to influence patient response to treatment.[16] However, severity of DO and voiding pattern did affect treatment outcome.

The long-term treatment with botulinum toxin in children was assessed by Schulte-Baukloh et al.[17] In total, 10 patients with NDO who had received at least three botulinum toxin injections, with mean age of 11.2 years at first injection, were reviewed. The outcomes 6 months after every other treatment, measured by urodynamics, were:

- increased reflex volume and bladder capacity
- decreased detrusor pressure
- increased bladder compliance.

Improved results were observed after repeat treatments, and no evidence of drug tolerance was noted.

Surgical therapy

Small intestine submucosal sling. Misseri and colleagues reviewed the outcomes of using small intestine submucosa (SIS) bladder-neck slings for treatment of incontinence associated with neuropathic bladder in the pediatric population.[18] A total of 21 girls and 15 boys (mean age 9 years) were treated with SIS bladder-neck slings with a mean follow-up of 15 months. Overall, 75% were dry following the sling procedure. The lowest success rate was noted in ambulatory boys with only 2 of 5 (40%) dry at follow-up.

Urethral closure. Stoffel and McGuire reported the outcome of urethral closure in patients with neurological impairment and complete urethral destruction.[19] All patients underwent urinary diversion. In total, 11 of 12 patients achieved continence at a median of 20 months; 5 patients required additional procedures to achieve this result. The authors concluded that, while surgical reconstruction in these patients presents a formidable challenge, persistence almost always results in continence.

Minimally invasive techniques. Mammen and Balaji reported the initial use of a surgical robotic system for detrusor myotomy as a minimally invasive surgical therapy for neurogenic bladder.[20]

Long-term follow-up of augmentation enterocystoplasty. Blaivas's group reviewed the long-term outcomes of 76 consecutive patients who underwent augmentation enterocystoplasty (AC) with or without an abdominal stoma.[21] The mean follow-up was 8.9 years. Of the 71 evaluable patients, 49 (69%) considered themselves cured, 14 (20%) considered themselves improved and 8 (11%) considered treatment to have failed. The overall long-term complication rate was 26.7%. The most common complications were related to the stoma (e.g. stomal stenosis and incontinence). Small-bowel obstruction and de novo bladder and renal stones were also seen.

Use of refluxing megaureters as Mitrofanoff channels. In a report of 35 patients requiring a Mitrofanoff continence procedure, Radojicic and colleagues proposed a variation using the distal end of a refluxing megaureter with simultaneous reimplantation of the proximal megaureter.[22] Minimal leakage occurred in 3 patients and was resolved with anticholinergics. This variant procedure expands the number of patients who may benefit from the use of the ureter for a Mitrofanoff channel.

Creation of a somatic–autonomic reflex pathway. Kelly et al. reported a novel technique for creation of a somatic–autonomic reflex pathway for the treatment of neurogenic bladder.[23] The goal of this procedure, which consists of L5 ventral root to S3 ventral root anastamosis, is to restore voluntary voiding in patients with suprasacral spinal cord injury (SCI). After the introduction of the technique in China, the first 2 patients who underwent this procedure in the USA were followed for 9 and 15 months. Cutaneous stimulation of the L5 root triggered detrusor contraction. Significant decreases in neurogenic overactivity on filling cystometry were observed with urodynamic assessment. One patient also reported improvement in bowel function. Follow-up studies are warranted. If this technique can be reproduced, it holds great promise for all kinds of impairments in patients with neurological disorders.

Highlights in **neurogenic bladder** *2005–06*

WHAT'S IN?

- Combination medical therapy with α-adrenergic and muscarinic antagonists to treat voiding dysfunction

- Tolerability and efficacy of trospium, darifenacin, solifenacin, and extended-release oxybutynin and tolterodine for neurogenic bladder

- Botulinum toxin types A and B for treatment options for neurogenic bladder and detrusor overactivity of neurogenic origin

- Neuromodulation

- Surgery for incontinence associated with neurogenic bladders

WHAT'S OUT?

- External sphincterotomy

- Single-modality therapy for neurogenic bladder

WHAT'S NEW?

- Non-invasive urodynamic evaluation

- Chronic pudendal nerve stimulation for refractory urinary urgency and frequency

- Surgical creation of somatic–autonomic reflex pathway for the treatment of neurogenic bladder due to spinal cord injury

- Robotic-assisted surgery for detrusor myotomy and augmentation cystoplasty

Neuromodulation

Application of neuromodulation to chronic pudendal nerve stimulation heralds a promising advance in the treatment of refractory urgency and frequency.

Peters et al. reported results of a prospective, single-blinded, randomized crossover trial of sacral (SNS) versus pudendal nerve stimulation (PNS) for refractory urgency, frequency and incontinence (n = 27) or neurogenic urinary retention (n = 3).[24] After a tined lead was placed at S3, all subjects had a second electrode placed at the pudendal nerve via a posterior approach. The pudendal nerve was confirmed with external anal sphincter needle electromyography. Both electrodes were externalized and patients were randomized to begin stimulation on either the sacral or pudendal nerve. Each lead was externalized and stimulated for 7 days in a blinded fashion. Patients subsequently selected which lead they preferred for permanent implantation. Overall, 24 of 30 patients were considered responders; 19 out of 24 chose the pudendal lead and only 5 out of 24 chose the sacral lead. Patients with PNS had superior subjective symptom improvement compared with that noted for SNS, but the two groups had almost identical improvements in objective voiding parameters.

Spinelli et al. described their series of 15 patients with neurogenic overactivity (8 male, 7 female) who underwent PNS via placement of a quadripolar tined lead near the pudendal nerve under neurophysiological guidance through a posterior or perineal approach.[25] A total of 8 patients became continent, and 4 were improved more than 50% in incontinence episodes. Of the 12 patients who continued to the second-stage implantation of the pulse generator, maximum cystometric capacity increased significantly at 6 months postoperatively. Longer-term follow-up is warranted.

References

1. Apostolidis A, Brady CM, Yiangou Y et al. Capsaicin receptor TRPV1 in urothelium of neurogenic human bladders and effect of intravesical resiniferatoxin. *Urology* 2005;65:400–5.

2. Apostolidis A, Popat R, Yiangou Y et al. Decreased sensory receptors P2X3 and TRPV1 in suburothelial nerve fibers following intradetrusor injections of botulinum toxin for human detrusor overactivity. *J Urol* 2005;174:977–82; discussion 982–3.

3. Giannantoni A, Di Stasi SM, Nardicchi V et al. Botulism A toxin intravesical treatment induces a reduction of nerve growth factor bladder tissue levels in patients with neurogenic detrusor overactivity. *J Urol* 2005;173(4 suppl):330(abstr 1217).

4. Gonzalez RR, Fong T, Belmar N et al. Modulating bladder neuroinflammation: RDP58, a novel anti-inflammatory peptide, reduces inflammation and nerve growth factor production in experimental cystitis. *J Urol* 2005;173:630–4.

5. Abdel-Karim AM, Barthlow HG, Bialecki RA, Elhilali MM. Effects of M274773, a neurokinin-2 receptor antagonist, on bladder function in chronically spinalized rats. *J Urol* 2005;174:1488–92.

6. Wuest M, Morgenstern K, Graf EM. Cholinergic and purinergic responses in isolated human detrusor in relation to age. *J Urol* 2005;173:2182–9.

7. Ahmed Y, Lin DL, Ferguson CL et al. Effects of estrogen on urethral function and molecular neuroregeneration after pudendal nerve injury in the female rat. *J Urol* 2005;173(4 suppl):251(abstr 928).

8. Griffiths CJ, Harding C, Blake C et al. A nomogram to classify men with lower urinary tract symptoms using urine flow and noninvasive measurement of bladder pressure. *J Urol* 2005;174:1323–6; discussion 1326; author reply 1326.

9. Nose H, Foo KT, Lim KB et al. Accuracy of two noninvasive methods of diagnosing bladder outlet obstruction using ultrasonography: intravesical prostatic protrusion and velocity-flow video urodynamics. *Urology* 2005;65:493–7.

10. Ruggieri MR Sr, Braverman AS, Pontari MA. Combined use of α-adrenergic and muscarinic antagonists for the treatment of voiding dysfunction. *J Urol* 2005;174:1743–8.

11. Ellsworth PI, Borgstein NG, Nijman RJ, Reddy PP. Use of tolterodine in children with neurogenic detrusor overactivity: relationship between dose and urodynamic response. *J Urol* 2005;174:1647–51; discussion 1651.

12. Franco I, Horowitz M, Grady R. Efficacy and safety of oxybutynin in children with detrusor hyperreflexia secondary to neurogenic bladder dysfunction. *J Urol* 2005;173:221–5.

13. Zinner N, Tuttle J, Marks L. Efficacy and tolerability of darifenacin, a muscarinic M3 selective receptor antagonist (M3 SRA), compared with oxybutynin in the treatment of patients with overactive bladder. *World J Urol* 2005;23:248–52.

14. Kelleher CJ, Cardozo L, Chapple CR et al. Improved quality of life in patients with overactive bladder symptoms treated with solifenacin. *BJU Int* 2005;95:81–5.

15. Schurch B, de Sèze M, Denys P et al.; Botox Detrusor Hyperreflexia Study Team. Botulinum toxin type A is a safe and effective treatment for neurogenic urinary incontinence: results of a single treatment, randomized, placebo controlled 6-month study. *J Urol* 2005;174: 196–200.

16. Schurch B, de Sèze M, Denys P et al. Botulism toxin A in neurogenic bladder: are there any patient predictors of response? *J Urol* 2005;173(4 suppl):305(abstr 1125).

17. Schulte-Baukloh H, Knispel HH, Stolze T et al. Repeated botulinum-A toxin injections in treatment of children with neurogenic detrusor overactivity. *Urology* 2005;66: 865–70; discussion 870.

18. Misseri R, Cain MP, Casale AJ et al. Small intestinal submucosa bladder neck slings for incontinence associated with neuropathic bladder. *J Urol* 2005;174:1680–2; discussion 1682.

19. Stoffel JT, McGuire EJ. Outcome of urethral closure in patients with neurologic impairment and complete urethral destruction. *Neurourol Urodyn* 2006;25:19–22.

20. Mammen T, Balaji KC. Robotic transperitoneal detrusor myotomy: description of a novel technique. *J Endourol* 2005;19:476–9.

21. Blaivas JG, Weiss JP, Desai P et al. Long-term followup of augmentation enterocystoplasty and continent diversion in patients with benign disease. *J Urol* 2005;173:1631–4.

22. Radojicic ZI, Perovic SV, Vukadinovic VM, Bumbasirevic MZ. Refluxing megaureter for the Mitrofanoff channel using continent extravesical detrusor tunneling procedure. *J Urol* 2005;174:693–5.

23. Kelly CE, Xiao CG, Weiner H et al. Creation of a somatic–autonomic reflex pathway for treatment of neurogenic bladder in patients with spinal cord injury: preliminary results of first 2 USA patients. *AUA Annual Meeting, 21–27 May 2005, San Antonio, TX, USA* 2005:abstr 1132. www.urotoday.com/search/contents/article.asp?cat=confReport&sid=184&tid=398&aid=3589

24. Peters KM, Feber KM, Konstandt D, Huynh PN. Sacral vs. pudendal nerve stimulation for voiding dysfunction: a prospective, single-blinded, randomized, crossover trial. *J Urol* 2005;173(4 suppl): 306(abstr 1127).

25. Spinelli M, Malaguti S, Giardiello G et al. A new minimally invasive procedure for pudendal nerve stimulation to treat neurogenic bladder: description of the method and preliminary data. *Neurourol Urodyn* 2005;24:305–9.

Female urology

Julian Shah FRCS

Institute of Urology and Nephrology, London, UK

Placement of tapes for the treatment of incontinence seems to be dominating the surgical intervention list. Some interesting papers on the pathophysiology of incontinence have been published, and evidence that cesarean section protects the pelvic floor continues to strengthen. We still need to determine whether the risks for mother and baby associated with cesarean section would be later outweighed by the morbidity associated with prolapse and incontinence and the subsequent risks and complications of surgery for these conditions.

Pathophysiological features of prolapse

The genes for proteins that relate to the extracellular matrix and intermediate filaments have been found to be overexpressed in cardinal ligament tissues in patients compared with controls.[1] The differential expression of these genes in patients may thus be risk markers for prolapse. Elastin fibers were thinner in patients with a large cystocele than in control patients. Aging also reduced elastin fiber width.[2] Fibroblast proliferation was lower in patients with prolapse than in control patients.[3] Genetic factors may also be at play in young women with prolapse who had a family history of prolapse and presented at a younger age (mean age 37 years) than the average (> 60 years).[4]

Vaginal delivery produces major effects on the levator ani. Levator ani avulsion occured in 36% of women who delivered vaginally,[5] an effect not seen in women who underwent cesarean section. Cesarean section was observed to have a protective effect on the pelvic floor.[6] However, the risks and benefits of vaginal compared with cesarean delivery have to be weighed up.

Aging

Bladder sensation decreases with age, along with detrusor strength and maximum urethral closure pressure. Bladder instability, however, increases sensitivity and reduces functional bladder capacity. Responses to anticholinergic medication may be different in the older woman for these reasons.[7] The overactive bladder can adversely affect the sexual quality of life in affected women.[8]

Fluid intake and incontinence

Patients with incontinence do not appear to reduce their daily fluid intake, contrary to popular belief.[9]

Exercise and incontinence

Women who experience urge incontinence are likely to exercise less. Thus, providing adequate treatment for these women would have definite benefits in terms of increasing physical activity, as well as in reducing troublesome symptoms.[10]

Ambulatory urodynamic studies

Once again it has been shown that ambulatory urodynamic studies are more effective than cystometry in diagnosing bladder instability. On ambulatory testing 64% of women were found to have instability, compared with only 25% found by cystometrogram. The test appears to be of less value in women with stress incontinence.[11]

Pelvic floor exercises

It is recommended that all women are offered pelvic floor exercises to treat stress urinary incontinence. Many patients will benefit in the early months, provided the exercises are performed regularly and support is offered. At 6 months, 60% of women were improved or dry after intensive therapy.[12] However, the benefits were not found to be maintained after 15 years had elapsed, many patients going on to have surgery for persistent incontinence.

Slings

Papers on the treatment of women with genuine stress incontinence (GSI) with slings continue to provide information about the longer-term outcomes and in particular the complications that are beginning to tax us (see below). New slings are also appearing on the market. Gynecare tension-free vaginal tape (TVT; Ethicon, Cornelia, GA, USA) was the first, but it now has many challengers. In particular, the transobturator tape (TOT) sling may overtake TVT as the primary surgical intervention for GSI.

Whether urodynamic studies should be performed before surgery for GSI remains controversial. Some clinicians believe that studies should be performed in all patients before surgery, whereas Sadiq and colleagues suggest that urodynamic studies are not necessary for women with GSI who have normal flow rates and residual volumes before surgery, as they found outcomes to be the same with or without urodynamics.[13]

The suprapubic arc (SPARC) synthetic sling system appears to carry similar success rate to other slings, with comparable risks and complications.[14]

In a comparison of the SPARC system with TOT (Monarc™, American Medical Systems, Minetonka, MN, USA), the outcome was the same in terms of resolution of stress incontinence and complication rate, suggesting that TOT is an attractive alternative to slings placed through the pelvis.[15] TOT (TVTO [TVT obturator]) was quicker to perform but had the same outcome as the TVT procedure (Gynecare), with similar success rates and complications.[16] Will TOT replace TVT? Thiel believes that it will.[17] He demonstrated that TOT (Porgès, Le Plessis Robinson, France) was quicker, easier, less complicated and better accepted. He also stated that TOT can be used after radiotherapy and previous pelvic surgery, which is a view that many of us hold. It is likely that this view will prevail in the next few years, provided that the long-term data from TOT uphold the claims made for this interesting procedure.

Adjusting the tension of a sling in order to avoid voiding dysfunction has been discussed on a number of occasions over the years and was certainly used, albeit sporadically, with the Stamey procedure. The SAFYRE sling (Promedon, Cordoba, Argentina) is adjustable in the postoperative period. In 200 women who underwent surgery with the SAFYRE sling, 20 required adjustment of the sling because of persistent incontinence, with 8 becoming dry and 4 improving. Complications appeared to be uncommon, as with other reports of sling procedures.[18]

In a comparison of porcine dermis (Pelvicol, Bard, Covington, GA, USA) and rectus sheath slings in two well-matched groups of women, clear advantages were observed for the latter.[19] The rectus sheath was associated with 80.4% cure rate for stress incontinence compared with 54% in the group who received porcine dermis slings.

Laparoscopic colposuspension is more expensive and less effective than the TVT procedure.[20]

Complications of slings. Although sling surgery is said to be minimally invasive and recovery swift, some aspects of life after surgery do not recover so quickly. Bakenga and colleagues showed that although most activities had returned to normal by 2 weeks, sporting activities, return to work and sexual activity took longer.[21]

Pelvic hematoma is one of the recognized complications of sling procedures. Magnetic resonance imaging showed that 25% of 24 patients had a retropubic hematoma after a sling procedure.[22] Irritable bladder symptoms after TVT may occur in up to 19% of women; patients should therefore be warned that these symptoms may persist in spite of resolution of stress incontinence.[23]

Hamilton Boyles and colleagues have estimated the complication rate following the TOT procedure. Few complications were reported, vaginal erosion and infection being the commonest (though still rare).[24] Bladder perforation was reported, but its true incidence is unknown, as cystoscopy is not performed routinely and there is controversy as to its role after the placement of the tape. It would seem appropriate that all women who undergo TOT placement should have a cystoscopy, which adds little to the time of the procedure.

Colposuspension

Equivalent results can be achieved during open or laparoscopic colposuspension by experienced surgeons, according to Smith and colleagues,[25] who also reported a discrepancy between subjective and objective outcomes in other studies of surgery for stress incontinence.

Artificial sphincters

The long-term benefits of the artificial urinary sphincter appear to be better in women than in men.[26] The first sphincter implants lasted for a median of 5 years in men, compared with 11.2 years in women. Women also experienced a higher continence rate.

Surgery for prolapse

Robots have been used to assist in the treatment of vaginal vault prolapse by laparoscopic colposacropexy and may provide benefits in both the surgical approach and in clinical recovery.[27] When compared with open surgery, laparoscopic surgery appears to have advantages in terms of less bleeding, less pain and shorter hospital stay.[28]

Urologic complications. Gustilo-Ashby and colleagues found an incidence of ureteric obstruction of 5.1% in 700 women who had undergone surgery for prolapse.[29] This is a higher incidence than one would initially expect and suggests that a high index of suspicion is necessary to ensure that this diagnosis is not missed.

Bladder instability – the overactive bladder

New medications for the management of this common and troublesome condition continue to come to market, solifenacin being the latest addition. A prospective double-blind, double-dummy study reported that solifenacin was superior to tolterodine.[30] However, patients do not appear to persist with anticholinergic treatment when it is prescribed for this troublesome condition. The most persistent cohort of patients in one study took their medication for a mean of 4.5 months.[31]

Sacral neuromodulation

For women with retention. Women with voiding dysfunction resulting from Fowler's syndrome are able to void with the assistance of sacral-nerve stimulation.[32] Voiding was maintained at a mean of 60 months by 63% of 30 patients. However, 23 of the 30 women required further intervention because of complications. The disease is difficult to manage and so this technique clearly has advantages; however, the complication rate is high and the long-term outcomes in this relatively young group of patients (mean age 33.7 years) are unknown at this stage.

Garne and colleagues showed neuromodulation to be effective in both overactive bladder and retention.[33] They assessed 23 patients, 14 of whom received implants; 11 of the patients (69%) were cured at a mean of 34.9 months.

For women with overactive bladder. In a double-blind, randomized study of trans-sacral stimulation, there was no difference between the treated and the sham-treated group.[34] In a small number of patients with a variety of symptoms, neuromodulation appeared to be effective in reducing urinary frequency, nocturia, urgency and voiding difficulty.[35]

Fistulas

Laparoscopic fistula repair has now been undertaken with success in a small number of patients and is suggested to offer excellent results with minimum morbidity.[36,37]

Bladders left after urinary diversion

Patients who undergo urinary diversion for a variety of non-malignant conditions often have the bladder left behind in order to reduce the morbidity of the procedure. What happens to the defunctionalized bladder? We have come to understand that about 25% of patients will develop pyocystis and require bladder removal. Fazili and colleagues showed that 54% of their 24 patients (mostly women) experienced problems with the retained bladder,[38] mostly infections. The Spence procedure was used in 3 of the 24 patients, with success in only 1; the bladder was removed in 6 patients.

Highlights in **female urology** 2005–06

WHAT'S IN?

- Ambulatory urodynamics for difficult cases
- Transobturator tape for stress incontinence
- Laparoscopic procedures, including robotic, for female disorders
- Cesarean section to prevent pelvic floor disorders and incontinence
- Autologous slings
- Anticholinergic medication and botulinum toxin for the unstable bladder (still)

WHAT'S OUT?

- Porcine dermis for slings

WHAT'S STILL IN BUT MAY BE ON THE WAY OUT?

- Tension-free vaginal tape
- Neuromodulation for the overactive bladder

These data confirm the problems associated with the retained bladder after diversion. However, large numbers of patients are spared cystectomy at the time of diversion, which must have benefits in terms of morbidity and mortality.

References

1. Liu M, Yip SK, Smith DI, Wong YF. Gene expression profiling of cardinal ligament in Hong Kong Chinese women with pelvic organ prolapse. *Neurourol Urodynam* 2005;24:425–6.

2. Zimmern P, Lin V, Sagalowsky A. Elastin in human prolapsed anterior vaginal wall of post-menopausal women. *Neurourol Urodynam* 2005; 24:426–7.

3. Liu YM, Choy KW, Lui WT et al. 17β-estradiol suppresses proliferation of fibroblasts derived from cardinal ligament in patients with or without pelvic organ prolapse (POP). *Neurourol Urodynam* 2005; 24:428–9.

4. Jack GS, Bukkapatnam R, Nicolav G et al. Autosomal dominant transmission of genitovaginal prolapse. *J Urol* 2005;173(4 suppl): 233–4.

5. Dietz HP, Lanzarone V. Vaginal delivery results in significant trauma to the levator ani muscle. *Neurourol Urodynam* 2005;24:509–10.

6. Lukacz E, Lawrence J, Nager C et al. The effect of pregnancy and mode of delivery on pelvic floor dysfunction: an epidemiologic study. *Neurourol Urodynam* 2005;24:508.

7. Pfisterer MH, Griffiths D, Schaefer W et al. The impact of aging and detrusor overactivity on female bladder function. *Neurourol Urodynam* 2005;24:456–7.

8. Rogers R, Margolis MK, Bavendam T et al. Overactive bladder with urinary incontinence adversely affects women's sexual quality. *J Urol* 2005;173(4 suppl):233–4.

9. Bryant C, Fairbrother G, Lloyd M. Fluid reduction behaviour among adults presenting for treatment with urinary incontinence/overactive bladder symptoms and a matched sample of controls. *Neurourol Urodynam* 2005;24:466–8.

10. Kinchen KS, Nygaard I, Fultz N et al. The impact of urinary incontinence on exercise. *J Urol* 2005;173(4 suppl):150.

11. Harding CK, Dorkin TJ, Leonard AS, Thorpe AC. The role of ambulatory urodynamic monitoring in the assessment of patients with incontinence. *BJU Int* 2005; 95(suppl 5):69.

12. Bo K, KvarsteinB, Nygaard I. Lower urinary tract symptoms 15 years after ending a randomised controlled trial of pelvic floor muscle training for urodynamic stress incontinence. *Eur Urol Suppl* 2005;4(3):91.

13. Sadiq A, Manunta A, Chograni S. TVT colposuspension without pre-operative urodynamic studies. *Eur Urol Suppl* 2005;4(3):15.

14. Gilling PJ, Benness C, Maxwell C. Australasian multi-centre study to evaluate the safety and efficacy of the SPARC sling procedure for female stress incontinence: results at one year. *BJU Int* 2005;95 (suppl 5):70.

15. Na TG, Youk SM, Kim YW. A prospective multicentre randomized study comparing transvaginal tapes (SPARC) and TOT suburethral tapes (Monarc) for the treatment of stress urinary incontinence. *Eur Urol Suppl* 2005;4(3):15.

16. Ryu KH, Shin JS, Choo MS, Lee KS. Randomized trial of tension-free vaginal tape (TVT) vs TVTO in the surgical treatment of stress urinary incontinence: comparison of operation related morbidity. *Eur Urol Suppl* 2005;4(3):15.

17. Thiel R. Retropubic vs transobturator approach (TVT vs TOT) for the treatment of stress incontinence. *Eur Urol Suppl* 2005;4(3):15.

18. Palma P, Riccetto C, Dambros M et al. Multicentric clinical study of a readjustable transobturator sling for female stress urinary incontinence. *Eur Urol Suppl* 2005;4(3):16.

19. Giri SK, Shaikh MF, McKenna P et al. Porcine dermis (Pelvicol™) vs rectus fascia pubovaginal sling in the treatment of stress incontinence: outcome analysis and patient satisfaction at a 3 year minimum follow-up. *BJU Int* 2005;95:71.

20. Valpas A, Rissanen P, Kujansuu E, Nilsson C. A cost-effectiveness analysis of tension free vaginal tape procedure vs laparoscopic mesh colposuspension for primary female stress incontinence – a randomized trial. *Neurourol Urodynam* 2005;24:418–19.

21. Bakenga J, Petrakian D, Irani J. Practical information to the patient before undergoing tension free vaginal tape (TVT) procedure. *Eur Urol Suppl* 2005;4(3):92.

22. Giri SK, Wallis F, Shaikh MF et al. Early haematoma formation and changes in pelvic anatomy following xenograft or tape sling: a prospective MRI-based study. *BJU Int* 2005;95:72.

23. Schraffordt S, Bisseling T, Heintz P et al. Changes in irritative bladder symptoms after TVT. A prospective multicentre 3 year follow-up study with the aid of the urogenital distress inventory (UDI-6) and incontinence impact questionnaire (IIQ-7). *Neurourol Urodynam* 2005;24:420–1.

24. Hamilton Boyles S, Gregory WT, Clark A, Edwards SR. Complications associated with trans-obturator sling procedures. *Neurourol Urodynam* 2005;24:423–5.

25. Smith A, Kitchener H, Dunne G et al. A prospective randomized controlled trial of open and laparoscopic colposuspension. *Neurourol Urodynam* 2005;24:422–3.

26. Petero VG, Diokno AC. Comparison of the long-term outcomes between incontinent men and women managed with artificial urinary sphincter. *J Urol* 2005;173:151.

27. Stoliar G, Corica FA, Sala LG et al. Initial experience with robotic-assisted laparoscopic sacrocolpopexy. *J Urol* 2005;173:233.

28. Hsaio KC, Kobashi KC, Govier FE, Kozlowski PM. Comparison of laparoscopic and open abdominal sacrocolpopexy. *J Urol* 2005;173:234.

29. Gustilo-Ashby AM, Jelovsek JE, Barber M. The incidence of ureteral obstruction and the value of intraoperative cystoscopy during vaginal surgery for pelvic organ prolapse. *Neurourol Urodynam* 2005;24:435.

30. Chapple C, Ballanger P, Hatzichristou D et al. Improvements in bladder condition in OAB as perceived and experienced by patients in a solifenacin vs tolterodine multinational study (STAR study). *Neurourol Urodynam* 2005;24:575.

31. Cisternas M, Noe L, Patel B et al. Comparison of persistence among therapies for overactive bladder: a retrospective pharmacy claims analysis. *Neurourol Urodynam* 2005;24:580–1.

32. Kavia RBC, Mishra V, Dasgupta R et al. Sacral neuromodulation for women with urinary retention: long-term results for the first 30 patients. *BJU Int* 2005;95(suppl 5):69.

33. Garne X, Sarramon JP, Mallet R. Results of sacral neuromodulation in neurogenic voiding dysfunction. *Eur Urol Suppl* 2005;4(3):165.

34. O'Reilly B, Achtari C, Hiscock R et al. A prospective randomized double-blind controlled trial evaluating the effect of trans-sacral magnetic stimulation in women with overactive bladder. *Neurourol Urodynam* 2005;24:489.

35. Gousse AE, Tunuguntla HSGR. Efficacy and safety of sacral neuromodulation in dysfunctional voiding of variable etiology. *J Urol* 2005;173(4 suppl):3.

36. Melamud O, Eichel L, Turbow B, Shamberg A. Robot-assisted laparoscopic vesico-vaginal fistula repair. *J Urol* 2005;173:134.

37. Sotelo RJ, Mariano MB et al. Vesico-vaginal fistula repair: our laparoscopic technique. *J Urol* 2005;173:134.

38. Fazili T, Bhat T, Khoriefs C et al. The fate of the "left over bladder" after supravesical urinary diversion. *BJU Int* 2005;95(suppl 5):41.

Erectile dysfunction

Ian Eardley MA MCHIR FRCS(Urol) FEBU

Department of Urology, St James' University Hospital, Leeds, UK

Epidemiology

Over the past decade there have been considerable advances in our understanding of the epidemiology of erectile dysfunction (ED). Much of this work has been supported by the pharmaceutical industry, but it has confirmed the prevalence of the condition and has clarified many of the disease associations, most notably the relationship between ED and cardiovascular disease. In 2005, there have been some new data relating to these associations, but of particular note have been the epidemiological studies that have explored (for the first time) the effects of erectile dysfunction upon the female partner.

The FEMALES study[1] questioned 293 female partners of men with ED. The onset of the ED was associated with a reduced frequency of sexual activity (as might be expected), but female desire, arousal and orgasm were also reduced. This is the first evidence that ED can be associated with an impairment of the female partner's sexual function. These changes correlated with the severity of the ED; there was also evidence that treatment of the man's ED with a phosphodiesterase type-5 (PDE5) inhibitor improved the sexual function of the female partner too.

ED and cardiovascular disease

The association between ED and cardiovascular disease has been long recognized and was elucidated further in 2005 with evidence of the association between ED, endothelial dysfunction and the metabolic syndrome. The definition of the metabolic syndrome has changed over the past few years, but the most recent recommendations of the International Diabetes Federation define the condition as the presence of central obesity (waist circumference greater than 94 cm for men) together with two of the following four factors:[2]

- raised serum triglyceride (≥ 1.7 mmol/L)
- reduced serum high-density lipoprotcin (HDL) cholesterol (< 1.03 mmol/L)
- raised blood pressure ($\geq 130/85$ mmHg)
- elevated fasting blood glucose (≥ 5.6 mmol/L).

In developed countries the prevalence of the metabolic syndrome is 22–39%, and its presence can predict cardiovascular morbidity. A study to explore the incidence in men presenting with ED showed that 43% of the entire cohort had evidence of the metabolic syndrome; when known diabetic men were excluded, the prevalence was 39%.[3] Insulin resistance was found in 79% of men, compared with a prevalence in the general population of about 25%. The converse of this study was undertaken in Naples, Italy, in 100 men with the metabolic syndrome matched with a control group. The prevalence of ED was found to be higher in the men with the metabolic syndrome (26.7% versus 13%, $p = 0.03$).[4]

In relation to the issue of cardiovascular risk factors, a recent epidemiological study clearly demonstrated an increased incidence of hypertension in 285 436 men with ED (41.2%) compared with 1 584 230 men without ED (19.2%).[5] Studies such as these emphasize the importance of correct investigation of men with ED, so that these cardiovascular risk factors can be identified and treated.

The appropriate assessment and treatment of men with proven cardiovascular disease was clearly defined in 2005. In 2000, the first Princeton Consensus Panel evaluated the degree of cardiovascular risk associated with sexual activity in men with cardiovascular disease.[6] The report of the second Princeton Consensus Panel was published in 2005[7] and clarified an algorithm for the assessment of such men, while emphasizing the importance of risk-factor evaluation and treatment for all men with ED. In short, at presentation, men with both ED and cardiovascular disease should be divided into one of three categories – low, intermediate or high cardiovascular risk. Men in the low-risk category can initiate or resume sexual activity and can be treated for sexual dysfunction without further cardiovascular investigation. Men at high risk should defer all sexual activity until the cardiac condition has been stabilized. Those in the intermediate-risk group should undergo cardiovascular assessment and restratification.

One particular group of men who, in the past, have been excluded from treatment with a PDE5 inhibitor are those using nitrates for ischemic heart disease. One paper published in 2005 suggested that this need not necessarily be so.[8] The authors optimized the cardiovascular therapy in a group of 88 men referred with ED who were using nitrates. They were able successfully to stop the nitrates in 49 of the men, allowing them to use the PDE5 inhibitor. The message is clear: if a man using nitrate medication is referred for treatment of ED, consideration should be given to stopping the nitrate so that a PDE5 inhibitor can be used. Inevitably, a cardiological opinion will be needed.

Medical therapy

First-line treatment for most men with ED continues to be an oral PDE5 inhibitor. Three medications are currently licensed: sildenafil, tadalafil and vardenafil. Numerous publications in 2005 defined the efficacy and safety of these three drugs, in particular, attempts to optimize treatment with PDE5 inhibitors and thereby minimize the number of patients in whom treatment fails.

Several studies have explored the treatment of men who have presented with self-reported failure of PDE5 inhibitor therapy.[9–11] It is clear from these studies that the physician must not assume that patients who have been referred with failure of PDE5 therapy have necessarily received an adequate trial of therapy with appropriate instructions on the use of the medication. Issues such as the need for appropriate sexual stimulation, awareness of the appropriate time window for the medication and avoidance of any food interactions are vital to maximize the chance of success. Furthermore, an adequate trial of therapy must include at least 6–8 attempts with the highest dose of the drug, since it has been clearly shown that several attempts are required to maximize the response rate to PDE5 inhibitors. It is also clear that alternative maneuvers can be tried, even when an adequate trial of a PDE5 inhibitor with sufficient, comprehensive instructions has failed. For instance, there is evidence that continuous daily dosing of a PDE5 inhibitor may be effective where intermittent usage has failed.[11,12] The mechanism behind this benefit is probably some generalized improvement in endothelial function.[13,14] Testosterone levels may modulate PDE5 expression and activity,[15] and it has been suggested that in men whose testosterone levels are low or in the lower end of the 'normal' range, testosterone supplementation might be effective.[16]

ED following radical prostatectomy

ED is one of the most frequent potential complications of radical retropubic prostatectomy (RRP) for localized prostate cancer. Numerous studies have suggested that predictors of postoperative erectile function include the patient's age, his preoperative erectile function, the presence of any preoperative risk factors for ED and the nerve-sparing status of the procedure. Erectile function may take up to 18 months to return, even in men in whom bilateral nerve sparing is achieved. In men who do develop ED, a number of mechanisms have been implicated, including unrecognized nerve injury, arterial injury and veno-occlusive dysfunction secondary to structural alterations in the cavernosal smooth muscle.

In 1997, Montorsi and colleagues proposed so-called rehabilitation as a means of preserving erectile function.[17] In a small prospective, randomized controlled trial, they demonstrated that early regular intracavernosal injections of prostaglandin E_1 (PGE_1) could help prevent ED. In a more recent randomized, placebo-controlled trial, it was demonstrated that, compared with placebo, regular nightly sildenafil resulted in a higher return of spontaneous erectile function 9 months after nerve-sparing RRP.[18] Mulhall and colleagues extended these findings, confirming the value of rehabilitation using a regimen of achieving at least three erections per week, by either oral pharmacotherapy with

Highlights in **erectile dysfunction** *2005–06*

WHAT'S IN?

- Awareness of the relationship between erectile dysfunction (ED), endothelial dysfunction and cardiovascular disease

- Optimization of oral phosphodiesterase type-5 (PDE5) inhibitor therapy

- Alternative strategies for men in whom standard PDE5 inhibitor therapy fails

WHAT'S NEW?

- New guidelines on the treatment of ED in men with cardiovascular disease

- Understanding of the effect of ED on female sexual function

- New protocols for the prevention of ED in men undergoing radical prostatectomy

- The possibility of gene therapy as a cure for ED

sildenafil or, if that was ineffective, intracavernosal PGE_1 injections.[19] In fact, most men in the rehabilitation group needed intracavernosal PGE_1 initially to achieve regular erections. However, the outcome of the trial suggested a clear advantage for the rehabilitation program, with 52% of men achieving spontaneous erections at 18 months, compared with 19% of those who were treated only as required ($p < 0.01$). If men who achieved erections in response to oral pharmacotherapy are included, the success rates for the two groups are 64% and 24%, respectively ($p < 0.01$). This trial confirms the value of such a rehabilitation program for men with ED following RRP, but further research will be needed to identify the optimal program.

New therapies

While PDE5 inhibitors remain first-line treatment for most men with ED, research continues into new methods of treatment. New drugs continue to be developed, and one that is attracting considerable interest is the melanocortin analog PT-141, which is administered intranasally. A study published in 2005, which used a RigiScan instrument (Osbon Medical Systems, Augusta, GA, USA), suggested that coadministration of PT-141 with sildenafil in men with ED might be more effective than either agent alone.[20]

Finally, research continues in the field of gene therapy. A group from New York has been at the forefront of investigation into the potential use of gene therapy as a means of curing ED and published the results of their first phase I trial in 2005.[21] They assessed the safety of a single injection of a plasmid vector that encoded for the high-conductance, calcium-activated potassium (maxi-K) channel of the cavernosal smooth muscle cell and were able to confirm that there were no adverse events. Research continues in this area.

References

1. Fisher WA, Rosen RC, Eardley I et al. Sexual experience of female partners of men with erectile dysfunction: The Female Experience of Men's Attitudes to Life Events and Sexuality (Females) study. *J Sex Med* 2005;2:677–84.

2. Alberti KG, Zimmet PZ, Shaw JE. The metabolic syndrome – a new worldwide definition. *Lancet* 2005;366:1059–60.

3. Bansal TC, Guay AT, Jacobsen J et al. Incidence of the metabolic syndrome and insulin resistance in a population with organic erectile dysfunction. *J Sex Med* 2005;2: 96–103.

4. Esposito K, Giugliano F, Martedi E et al. High proportions of erectile dysfunction in men with the metabolic syndrome. *Diabetes Care* 2005;28:1201–3.

5. Sun P, Swindle R. Are men with erectile dysfunction more likely to have hypertension than men without erectile dysfunction? *J Urol* 2005; 174:244–9.

6. DeBusk R, Drory Y, Goldstein I et al. Management of sexual dysfunction in patients with cardiovascular disease: recommendations of The Princeton Consensus Panel. *Am J Cardiol* 2000;86:175–81.

7. Kostis JB, Jackson G, Rosen R et al. Sexual dysfunction and cardiac risk (the Second Princeton Consensus Conference). *Am J Cardiol* 2005;96: 313–21.

8. Jackson G, Martin E, McGing E, Cooper A. Successful withdrawal of oral long-acting nitrates to facilitate phosphodiesterase type 5 inhibitor use in stable coronary disease patients with erectile dysfunction. *J Sex Med* 2005;2:513–16.

9. Hatzichristou DG, Moysidis K, Apostolidis A et al. Sildenafil failures may be due to inadequate patient instructions and follow-up: a study of 100 non-responders. *Eur Urol* 2005;47:518–22.

10. Gruenwald I, Shenfield O, Chen J et al. Positive effect of counselling and dose adjustment in patients with erectile dysfunction who failed treatment with sildenafil. *Eur Urol* 2006;49: in press.

11. Hatzimouratidis K, Moysidis K, Bekos A et al. Treatment strategy for "Non-responders" to tadalafil and vardenafil. A real life study. *Eur Urol* 2006;49: in press.

12. McMahon C. Efficacy and safety of daily tadalafil in men with erectile dysfunction previously unresponsive to on-demand tadalafil. *J Sex Med* 2004;1:292–300.

13. Katz SD, Balidemaj K, Homma S et al. Acute type 5 phosphodiesterase inhibition with sildenafil enhances flow mediated vasodilation in patients with chronic heart failure. *J Am Coll Cardiol* 2000;36:845–51.

14. Rosano GM, Aversa A, Vitale C et al. Chronic treatment with tadalafil improves endothelial function in men with increased cardiovascular risk. *Eur Urol* 2005;47:214–20.

15. Morelli A, Filippi S, Mancina R et al. Androgens regulate phosphodiesterase type 5 expression and functional activity in corpora cavernosa. *Endocrinology* 2004;145: 2253–63.

16. Shabsigh R, Kaufman JM, Steidle C, Padma-Nathan H. Randomized study of testosterone gel as adjunctive therapy to sildenafil in hypogonadal men with erectile dysfunction who do not respond to sildenafil alone. *J Urol* 2004;172:658–63.

17. Montorsi F, Gnazzoni G, Strambi LF et al. Recovery of spontaneous erectile function after nerve sparing radical retropubic prostatectomy with and without early intracavernous injections of alprostadil: results of a prospective, randomised trial. *J Urol* 1997;158:1408–10.

18. Padma-Nathan H, McCullough AR, Giuliano F et al. Postoperative nightly administration of sildenafil citrate significantly improves the return of normal spontaneous erectile function after bilateral nerve-sparing radical prostatectomy. *J Urol* 2003:169(suppl):375–6(A1402).

19. Mulhall J, Land S, Parker M et al. The use of an erectogenic pharmacotherapy regimen following radical prostatectomy improves recovery of spontaneous erectile function. *J Sex Med* 2005;2:532–42.

20. Diamond LE, Earle DC, Garcia WD, Spana C. Co-administration of low doses of intra-nasal PT-141, a melanocortin receptor agonist, and sildenafil to men with erectile dysfunction results in an enhanced erectile response. *Urology* 2005;65:755–9.

21. Melman A, Bar-Chama N, McCullough A et al. The first human trial for gene transfer therapy for the treatment of erectile dysfunction: preliminary results. *Eur Urol* 2005; 48:314–18.

Benign prostatic hyperplasia

Eva DM Fong MBChB and Peter J Gilling FRACS (Urol)
Promed Urology, Tauranga, New Zealand

Comorbidities and etiology

In the last year further interest in diseases associated with benign prostatic hyperplasia (BPH) has centered on autonomic dysfunction, vascular disease, erectile dysfunction, prostatitis and renal failure.

McVary and colleagues studied a subset of 38 patients from the Medical Treatment of Prostatic Symptoms (MTOPS) trial with tilt table and catecholamine testing.[1] In this study there was a strong association between autonomic activity and measures of BPH (American Urological Association BPH index scores and prostate volume).

Nickel et al. evaluated 608 men who complained of painful ejaculation from a total of 3700 BPH patients (in the ALF-ONE trial).[2] Men in this subgroup were more likely than others to report severe lower urinary tract symptoms (LUTS) and bother, erectile dysfunction, history of urinary tract infection (UTI) and macroscopic hematuria. The authors suggested more evaluation and treatment strategies were needed to target patients with both BPH and prostatitis-like symptoms.

Berger and colleagues investigated vascular damage as a common risk factor for BPH and erectile dysfunction.[3] Using contrast-enhanced Doppler ultrasonography they demonstrated diminished perfusion of the prostatic transition zone in non-diabetic and diabetic patients with BPH compared with healthy controls. Mean arterial flow in the corpora cavernosa was slower in diabetic than in non-diabetic patients with BPH; both were slower than controls. These findings suggest that ischemia is a common etiologic factor in both BPH and erectile dysfunction.

Rule et al. reviewed the medical literature from 1966 to 2003 to determine whether BPH is a causative factor for renal failure.[4]

Combinations of chronic retention with large residual urine volumes (greater than 300 mL), detrusor instability and decreased bladder compliance were associated with chronic renal failure (CRF). Ureterovesicular junction obstruction from bladder remodeling in chronic urinary retention was the most commonly proposed mechanism for CRF, perhaps with episodic acute urinary retention, urinary tract infections and secondary hypertension also contributing. Studies showed significant improvement in renal function after prostate surgery. They demonstrated that there is a strong association, probably causal, with further large community-based studies needed to confirm this.

Molecular biology

Research in this area has focused on development of models of cell–cell and stromal–cell interaction to study further the complex interactions which lead to BPH.[5] Shariat and colleagues demonstrated upregulation of survivin expression that correlated with International Prostate Symptom Score (IPSS), quality of life, post-void residual volume (PVR) and flow rate, suggesting that an increase in proliferation and inhibition of apoptosis has a role in BPH.[6]

Vela-Navarrete et al. demonstrated that an extract of saw palmetto significantly increased the *Bax*-to-*Bcl-2* ratio, a measure of apoptosis.[7]

Natural history

Further data on the natural history of LUTS following treatment have been published by Thomas et al.,[8] who followed 217 men for at least 13 years after transurethral resection of the prostate (TURP). The patients generally had sustained symptomatic improvement long-term. When failed patients were analyzed by urodynamic diagnosis and stratified by maximum urinary flow (Q_{max}), those in the significantly impaired group (< 10 mL/s) were equally likely to have bladder outlet obstruction (30%) or detrusor failure (43%). Cases of slightly better flow (Q_{max} 10–15 mL/s) were principally associated with detrusor failure. This study suggests that

53

patients who fail after TURP need urodynamic investigation to identify the cause, likely to be detrusor failure rather than recurrent bladder outlet obstruction in a significant proportion of patients.

Two studies have examined the natural history of community-dwelling men with respect to LUTS. Roberts and colleagues described the limitations of using the placebo arm of a BPH trial to represent community-based men, showing that there were lower rates of symptoms and progression in the placebo arm of the MTOPS trial than in community-dwelling men.[9]

Rule et al. followed 529 community-dwelling men with PVR and voided volume measurements every 2 years for 12 years. They found progressive bladder dysfunction with age in community-dwelling men. Signs and symptoms attributed to BPH were modest predictors of the development of bladder dysfunction; however, an increased PVR predicted a rapid decrease in voided volume, consistent with a bladder outlet obstruction contributing to the development of detrusor overactivity and decreased bladder compliance.[10]

Medical therapy

The impact of medical therapy on surgical management over a decade (1992–2002) was examined by Vela-Navarrete et al.[11] Over this period there was a 17.6% decrease in patients having surgery; those who did have surgery were an average of 3.1 years older and had received a longer period of medical treatment beforehand. However, indications for surgery were similar across the decade.

α-blockers. Interest in α-blocker medications has centered on side effects, sexual dysfunction and combination therapy with other medications.

Zlotta et al. surveyed 2511 patients participating in three double-blind, randomized trials who were taking Permixon (a phyto-therapeutic agent from the saw palmetto, *Serenoa repens*), tamsulosin or finasteride about their sexual function.[12] There was a difference at 6 months with increased sexual disorders (mostly ejaculation disorders) with tamsulosin and finasteride but not with Permixon.

Chang and colleagues described the floppy iris syndrome as a side effect of tamsulosin.[13] The phenomenon referred to is a triad of billowing of the flaccid iris stroma, progressive pupil constriction during surgery and propensity for iris prolapse at the time of cataract surgery. This occurred in 2% of 511 patients, all of whom were receiving tamsulosin. A review by Lawrentschuk and Bylsma gives 'a urologist's guide' to this problem.[14] They cite several problems with diagnostic criteria and sensitivity while acknowledging the strong statistical association demonstrated by Chang. They recommend no change in prescribing practices based on a single early report but suggest practical measures including asking patients if they have cataracts and will undergo surgery, instructing patients to inform their ophthalmologist that they are taking tamsulosin and discontinuing use of tamsulosin 7 days prior to surgery. This area requires further investigation as there is insufficient evidence on the length of tamsulosin discontinuation that will guarantee a reduced risk of floppy iris syndrome.

Combination therapy continues to be studied to try to improve the success of medical management. Lee et al. investigated combined therapy with anticholinergics and α-blockers (using propiverine hydrochloride plus doxazosin controlled-release gastrointestinal therapeutic system formulation) in a randomized multicenter trial of 211 patients.[15] They found that although PVR and adverse events were increased in the combination group, there was no difference in urinary retention overall or withdrawal from treatment. Both groups had improved flow rates and IPSS scores, with the combination group having greater improvement rates with regard to urinary frequency, average micturition volume and storage and urgency.

α-reductase inhibitors. The effects of the 5α-reductase inhibitor dutasteride were assessed for durability at 4 years, showing sustained decreases in IPSS and increase in flow rate.[16]

Surgical treatments
Microwave therapy. A number of medium-term trial outcomes have been published in the last year.

Wagrell et al. published a 36-month update of their outcomes from a prospective randomized trial of microwave therapy versus TURP.[17] They showed that TURP was superior in decreasing IPSS at 36 months and Q_{max} at 12 months; however, quality of life and Q_{max} were not significantly different between the groups at 36 months. Adverse effects described as serious were reported in 2% of microwave and 17% of TURP patients.

Walmsley and Kaplan reviewed the status of microwave thermotherapy in October 2004, commenting that the effects of treatment appeared to be durable; however, the re-treatment rates were significantly higher than those for TURP, 20–25% versus 5% at 5 years.[18]

Laser. During the past year further data have become available describing the outcomes of KTP (potassium titanyl phosphate) laser treatment and holmium laser enucleation of the prostate (HoLEP); other wavelengths are used less often.

KTP laser therapy. Short-term (6-month) direct comparison between KTP and TURP has been described by Bachmann,[19] with similar changes in IPSS and Q_{max} and similar complication rates (although different types of events).

Malek et al. reported 5-year follow-up of 94 patients treated with KTP.[20] However, since the acquisition of patients was incremental over that time, only 24 patients had matured to 5 years and only 14 of these were evaluable. In their cohort virtually all patients had at least a 50% improvement in their IPSS score and most had improvement in flow rate at 5 years. This study reported no serious adverse effects, notably no incontinence or impotence.

Several authors have reported using KTP for specific clinical applications, namely large prostates and anticoagulated patients. Sandhu and colleagues reported experience with large prostates (mean 100 mL).[21] They also reported anticoagulated patients,[22] as did Reich et al.[23] In all studies no transfusion was required, despite continuation of aspirin and clopidogrel or only brief discontinuation (2 days) of warfarin. Improvements in IPSS and Q_{max} were comparable to other KTP studies.

HoLEP has been further examined, both by studies in specific clinical scenarios (acute retention, the outpatient setting and large prostate size) and in direct comparison to TURP and bladder neck incision.

Peterson et al.[24] and Elzayat et al.[25] reviewed 164 and 169 patients, respectively, who had undergone HoLEP for acute urinary retention. Despite large prostate size (mean 107.1 and 101 mL), all but 3 patients reported by the Elzayat group were able to void satisfactorily postoperatively with similar transfusion rates and catheter times to those in previous HoLEP studies.

Elzayat further examined HoLEP in large glands (mean 82.7 mL), showing 200% improvement in Q_{max} and 75% improvement in IPSS.[26]

Aho and colleagues examined outpatient surgery with HoLEP versus holmium laser bladder-neck incision (HoBNI) in a randomized controlled trial in prostates of size less than 40 g.[27] They showed that HoBNI was associated with significant failure in prostates larger than 30 g, 5 out of 20 having obstruction at 6 months necessitating HoLEP. HoLEP was successfully employed on an outpatient basis in this patient group.

Two further randomized studies by Kuntz et al.[28] and Montorsi et al.[29] compared HoLEP and TURP. These studies included 200 and 100 patients, respectively, with follow-up to 1 year. They found that HoLEP was at least as effective as TURP for relieving obstruction and LUTS. Montorsi found no significant difference in flow rate and IPSS at 12 months, whereas Kuntz found that HoLEP was superior in both parameters. In both studies transfusion rates, hospital stay and catheter time were less for HoLEP; however, sexual dysfunction, including retrograde ejaculation, was similar.

Tinmouth and colleagues reviewed 509 cases, and found that prostate-specific antigen (PSA) diminution correlated with resected adenoma weight and with change in volume by transrectal ultrasound; they suggested that the decrease in PSA may be a surrogate for tissue removal.[30] This important study has implications for treatments in which no tissue is retrieved, such as ablation.

Other technologies. Administration of botulinum toxin by the transperineal route has been reported. Kuo reported the first transurethral prostatic injection in 10 patients who were poor surgical candidates.[31] His study produced significant improvement in flow rate and, interestingly, given concerns about the transient effects of this treatment, was the first study to demonstrate further improvement between 3 and 6 months after treatment.

The use of laparoscopic adenomectomy in BPH has been reported by Sotelo et al.,[32] Rehman et al.[33] and Rey et al.[34] Rey and colleagues performed 20 cases using both transvesical and Millin techniques and described the first two cases followed up for longer than a year. Adenoma tissue of masses 138 g and 102 g was removed with operative times of 120 and 180 minutes, respectively, and acceptable blood loss.

Transurethral resection of the prostate. Competing technologies have led to an emphasis on reducing the morbidity of TURP.

Singh et al. randomized 60 patients to bipolar or monopolar TURP.[35] They found that there was no difference in resected tissue amount, irrigant amount, fluid absorption, duration and amount of postoperative irrigation and fall in hemoglobin. There were similar improvements in urine flow and symptom scores. In the bipolar group, however, the fall in serum sodium was smaller and postoperative dysuria was less.

Sciarra et al. conducted a trial on 96 patients with cyclooxygenase-2 (COX-2) inhibitors versus no treatment to reduce urethral stricture after TURP.[36] After TURP, COX-2 inhibitors were commenced at catheter removal for a course of 20 days. The authors found a significant difference in stricture rate at 1 year: 17% in the untreated group versus 0% in the COX-2 group. This treatment clearly warrants further investigation.

Ghalayini and colleagues questioned whether a period of clean intermittent self-catheterization before TURP would improve bladder function and therefore surgical outcomes.[37] In total, 41 patients with similar pretreatment parameters, including PVR greater than 300 mL, were randomized to either clean intermittent

Highlights in **benign prostatic hyperplasia 2005–06**

WHAT'S IN?

- Urodynamic investigation in patients who fail transurethral resection of the prostate (TURP) to identify the cause

- Holmium laser enucleation of the prostate, potassium titanyl phosphate (KTP) laser therapy and saline (bipolar) TURP

- PSA reduction as a surrogate for tissue removal in BPH therapies

- The role of inflammation in BPH progression

- Investigation and treatment of concomitant disorders such as vascular and inflammatory diseases (e.g. prostatitis)

- Randomized controlled trials as evidence for new therapies

WHAT'S OUT?

- Using the placebo arm of a BPH trial to represent community-based men

- Accepting morbidity from TURP

- Reimbursement-driven treatment options

WHAT'S NEEDED?

- Randomized controlled trials of KTP laser ablation

- More evidence on the association between tamsulosin and floppy iris syndrome

- More research on the association between BPH and renal failure

self-catheterization or TURP. Both groups showed improved IPSS and quality-of-life parameters. In the self-catheterization group there was a significant improvement in voiding and end-filling pressures, indicating recovery of bladder function.

The future

New therapies are directed towards the static component of BPH, namely metabolic factors (hexokinase inhibitors), growth factors (vitamin D_3 analogs), oxytocin antagonists and gonadotropin-releasing hormone Gi agonist-based therapies.[38] Future work is also likely to address the role of inflammation in BPH, demonstrated in basic science and early clinical studies, as a target for therapy.

References

1. McVary KT, Rademaker A, Lloyd G, Gann P. Autonomic nervous system overactivity in men with lower urinary tract symptoms secondary to benign prostatic hyperplasia. *J Urol* 2005;174;1327–33.

2. Nickel JC, Elhilali M, Vallancien G; ALF-ONE Study Group. Benign prostatic hyperplasia (BPH) and prostatitis: prevalence of painful ejaculation in men with clinical BPH. *BJU Int* 2005;95:571–4.

3. Berger AP, Deibl M, Leonhartsberger N et al. Vascular damage as a risk factor for benign prostatic hyperplasia and erectile dysfunction. *BJU Int* 2005;96:1073–8.

4. Rule AD, Lieber MM, Jacobsen SJ. Is benign prostatic hyperplasia a risk factor for chronic renal failure? *J Urol* 2005;173:691–6.

5. Barclay W, Woodruff R, Hall C, Cramer S. A system for studying epithelial–stromal interactions reveals distinct inductive abilities of stromal cells from benign prostatic hyperplasia and prostate cancer. *Endocrinology* 2005;146:13–28.

6. Shariat S, Ashfaw R, Roehrborn CG et al. Expression of surviving and apoptotic biomarkers in benign prostatic hyperplasia. *J Urol* 2005;174:2046–50.

7. Vela-Navarrete R, Escribano-Burgos M, López Farré A et al. *Serenoa repens* treatment modifies *bax/bcl-2* index expression and caspase-3 activity in prostatic tissue from patients with benign prostatic hyperplasia. *J Urol* 2005;173: 507–10.

8. Thomas AW, Cannon A, Bartlett E et al. The natural history of lower urinary tract dysfunction in men: minimum 10-year urodynamic followup of transurethral resection of prostate for bladder outlet obstruction. *J Urol* 2005;174: 1887–91.

9. Roberts RO, Lieber MM, Jacobson DJ et al. Limitations of using outcomes in the placebo arm of a clinical trial of benign prostatic hyperplasia to quantify those in the community. *Mayo Clin Proc* 2005;80:759–64.

10. Rule AD, Jacobson DJ, McGree ME et al. Longitudinal changes in post-void residual and voided volume among community dwelling men. *J Urol* 2005;174: 1317–22.

11. Vela-Navarrete R, Gonzalez-Enguita C, Garcia-Cardoso JV et al. The impact of medical therapy on surgery for benign prostatic hyperplasia: a study comparing changes in a decade (1992–2002). *BJU Int* 2005;96:1045–8.

12. Zlotta AR, Teillac P, Raynaud JP, Schulman CC. Evaluation of male sexual function in patients with lower urinary tract symptoms (LUTS) associated with benign prostatic hyperplasia (BPH) treated with a phytotherapeutic agent (Permixon®), tamsulosin or finasteride. *Eur Urol* 2005;48:269–76.

13. Chang DF, Campbell JR. Intraoperative floppy iris syndrome associated with tamsulosin. *J Cataract Refract Surg* 2005;31:664–73.

14. Lawrentschuk N, Bylsma G. Intraoperative 'floppy iris' syndrome and its relationship to tamsulosin: a urologist's guide. *BJU Int* 2006;97: 2–3.

15. Lee KS, Choo MS, Kim DY et al. Combination treatment with propiverine hydrochloride plus doxazosin controlled release gastrointestinal therapeutic system formulation for overactive bladder and coexisting benign prostatic obstruction: a prospective, randomized, controlled multicenter study. *J Urol* 2005;174:1334–8.

16. Roehrborn CG, Lukkarinen O, Mark S et al. Long-term sustained improvement in symptoms of benign prostatic hyperplasia with the dual 5α-reductase inhibitor dutasteride: results of 4-year studies. *BJU Int* 2005;96:572–7.

17. Wagrell L, Schelin S, Nordling J et al. Three-year follow-up of feedback microwave thermotherapy versus TURP for clinical BPH: a prospective randomized multicenter study. *Urology* 2004;64:698–702.

18. Walmsley K, Kaplan SA. Transurethral microwave thermotherapy for benign prostate hyperplasia: separating truth from marketing hype. *J Urol* 2004;172: 1249–55.

19. Bachmann A, Schurch L, Ruszat R et al. Photoselective vaporization (PVP) versus transurethral resection of the prostate (TURP): a prospective bi-centre study of perioperative morbidity and early functional outcome. *Eur Urol* 2005;48:965–71.

20. Malek RS, Kuntzman RS, Barrett DM. Photoselective potassium-titanyl-phosphate laser vaporization of the benign obstructive prostate: observations on long-term outcomes. *J Urol* 2005;174:1344–8.

21. Sandhu JS, Ng C, Vanderbrink BA et al. High-power potassium-titanyl-phosphate photoselective laser vaporization of prostate for treatment of benign prostatic hyperplasia in men with large prostates. *Urology* 2004;64:1155–9.

22. Sandhu JS, Ng CK, Gonzalez RR et al. Photoselective laser vaporization prostatectomy in men receiving anticoagulants. *J Endourol* 2005;19:1196–8.

23. Reich O, Bachmann A, Siebels M. High power (80 W) potassium-titanyl-phosphate laser vaporization of the prostate in 66 high risk patients. *J Urol* 2005;173:158–60.

24. Peterson MD, Matlaga BR, Kim SC et al. Holmium laser enucleation of the prostate for men with urinary retention. *J Urol* 2005;174:998–1001; discussion 1001.

25. Elzayat EA, Habib EI, Elhilali MM. Holmium laser enucleation of prostate for patients in urinary retention. *Urology* 2005;66:789–93.

26. Elzayat EA, Habib EI, Elhilali MM. Holmium laser enucleation of the prostate: a size-independent new "gold standard". *Urology* 2005; 66(5 suppl 1):108–13.

27. Aho TF, Gilling PJ, Kennett KM et al. Holmium laser bladder neck incision versus holmium enucleation of the prostate as outpatient procedures for prostates less than 40 grams: a randomized trial. *J Urol* 2005;174:210–14.

28. Kuntz RM, Ahyai S, Lehrich K, Fayad A. Transurethral holmium laser enucleation of the prostate versus transurethral electrocautery resection of the prostate: a randomized prospective trial in 200 patients. *J Urol* 2004;172:1012–16.

29. Montorsi F, Naspro R, Salonia A et al. Holmium laser enucleation versus transurethral resection of the prostate: results from a 2-center, prospective, randomized trial in patients with obstructive benign prostatic hyperplasia. *J Urol* 2004;172:1926–9.

30. Tinmouth WW, Habib E, Kim SC et al. Change in serum prostate specific antigen concentration after holmium laser enucleation of the prostate: a marker for completeness of adenoma resection? *J Endourol* 2005;19:550–4.

31. Kuo HC. Prostate botulinum A toxin injection – an alternative treatment for benign prostatic obstruction in poor surgical candidates. *Urology* 2005;65:670–4.

32. Sotelo R, Spaliviero M, Garcia-Segui A et al. Laparoscopic retropubic simple prostatectomy. *J Urol* 2005;173:757–60.

33. Rehman J, Khan SA, Sukkarieh T et al. Extraperitoneal laparoscopic prostatectomy (adenomectomy) for obstructing benign prostatic hyperplasia: transvesical and transcapsular (Millin) techniques. *J Endourol* 2005;19:491–6.

34. Rey D, Ducarme G, Hoepffner JL, Staerman F. Laparoscopic adenectomy: a novel technique for managing benign prostatic hyperplasia. *BJU Int* 2005;95:676–8.

35. Singh H, Desai M, Shrivastav P, Vani K. Bipolar versus monopolar transurethral resection of prostate: randomized controlled study. *J Endourol* 2005;19:333–8.

36. Sciarra A, Salciccia S, Albanesi L et al. Use of cyclooxygenase-2 inhibitor for prevention of urethral strictures secondary to transurethral resection of the prostate. *Urology* 2005;66:1218–22.

37. Ghalayini I, Al-Gahzo M, Pickard R. A prospective randomized trial comparing transurethral prostatic resection and clean intermittent self-catheterization in men with chronic urinary retention. *BJU Int* 2005;96:93–7.

38. Tiwari A, Krishna NS, Nanda K, Chugh A. Benign prostatic hyperplasia: an insight into current investigational medical therapies. *Expert Opin Investig Drugs* 2005;14:1359–72.

Prostate cancer

Alexandre R Zlotta MD and Claude Schulman MD PhD
Department of Urology, Erasme Hospital, University Clinics of Brussels, Brussels, Belgium

Effects of long-term vitamin E supplementation on cardiovascular events and cancer

The potential chemopreventive effect of vitamin E on prostate cancer has been hypothesized for a couple of years. A randomized, double-blind, placebo-controlled international trial that enrolled 9541 patients examined the usefulness of vitamin E, 400 IU, on cardiovascular and cancer risk. At 7-year follow-up, this trial showed no beneficial effect of vitamin E in reducing the occurrence of any cancer and in particular in reducing prostate cancer incidence or mortality.[1] Moreover, an increased risk of heart failure was observed in the intervention arm!

Cancers detected at the third round of the ERSSPC

The Finnish trial, with approximately 80 000 men in the target population, is the largest component in the European Randomized Study of Screening for Prostate Cancer (ERSSPC). The first round was completed in 1996–1999. Each year, 8000 men aged 55–67 years were randomly assigned to the screening arm, and the rest formed the control arm. The screening interval was 4 years. Of the eligible men, 69% participated in the second round of screening, giving a detection rate of 2.1%.

In the third round, prostate cancer was detected in 2.9% of 213 patients who were screened positive for prostate-specific antigen (PSA). Interestingly, 75% of the men with prostate cancer had a Gleason score below 6, raising the question as to whether these small, well-differentiated tumors should be detected.[2]

Prostate-specific antigen testing

Initial PSA values and subsequent risk of prostate cancer. Baseline
PSA levels and future prostate cancer risk has been evaluated from
data from the randomized Swedish arm of the ongoing ERSSPC.
None of the men who, 10 years ago, had PSA values in the range
0–0.4 ng/mL developed prostate cancer. The risk increased to 25%
if baseline PSA levels were between 2.5 and 2.9 ng/mL.[3]

Is additional testing necessary in men with PSA below 1.0 ng/mL?
Data from the Prostate Cancer Prevention Trial (PCPT) have shown
that even at very low PSA levels, the risk of undetected prostate
cancer, although low, is not zero. In the ERSSPC, with a totally
different design from the PCPT and a different patient population,
data show a very low yield for diagnostic procedures at these very
low PSA levels. Indeed, in 1703 men aged 55–65 years with an
initial PSA level of 1.0 ng/mL or lower, 2344 subsequent PSA
determinations in an 8-year period after the initial screening resulted
in detection of eight cancers, giving a dismal overall cancer
detection rate of 0.47%. A strategy of PSA screening every 8 years
for men with a PSA level of 1.0 ng/mL or less may thus reduce the
number of screening visits (with the associated costs and stress),
with a minimal risk of missing aggressive cancer.[4]

Lower PSA levels in obese men. A population-based study of
2779 men without prostate carcinoma found that mean PSA
values decrease with increase in body mass index. Lower PSA
levels in obese men could thus mask a sign of prostate cancer.[5]
   Interestingly, a strong association between obesity and
biochemical progression after radical prostatectomy was also
observed among men treated in the last 10 years.[6]

**Characteristics of cancers found at low initial PSA levels
(below 3 ng/mL).** The highly publicized PCPT has already drawn
attention to the limits of PSA as a diagnostic marker for prostate
cancer. A total of 1225 cancers were found in the subset of
8575 patients who initially had a PSA level of no more than

3 ng/mL. Over 20% had a Gleason score of 7, and an additional 5% of cases had a Gleason score of 8 or higher, accounting for more than 25% of cases of aggressive disease.

There was no cut-off value for PSA levels that had both high sensitivity and high specificity for detecting prostate cancer in healthy men, but rather a continuum of prostate cancer risk at all PSA values.[7]

Pretreatment PSA velocity above 2 ng/mL/year has previously been shown to be associated with a highly significant increase in prostate-cancer-specific mortality despite radical surgery.

Another study of 202 men who underwent surgery has also shown that disease-free survival at 5 years was significantly lower if PSA velocity before surgery was above 2 ng/mL/year (73 vs 89%). Patients with PSA velocity above 2 ng/mL/year were more likely to harbor pT3 disease, positive margins and grade 4/5 tumors.[8]

PSA velocity is also an important prognostic factor in patients treated with radiation therapy. In 358 men treated with radiation for localized prostate cancer, PSA velocity above 2 ng/mL/year before therapy was associated with a significantly shorter time to prostate-cancer-specific and all-cause mortality.[9]

These results stress the importance of determining PSA kinetics before radiotherapy even in men with localized disease.

Prostate-cancer-specific mortality after PSA recurrence. In 379 men treated with radical prostatectomy and followed up for a mean duration of 10 years, PSA doubling time (< 3, 3–8.9, 9–14.9, > 15 months), Gleason score (≤ 7 or 8–10) and time to PSA recurrence after surgery (≤ 3 or > 3 years) were all significant risk factors for time to prostate-cancer-specific mortality.[10] Median survival in this cohort of patients had not been reached in 16 years of follow-up after PSA recurrence.

Similarly, PSA doubling times of less than 3 months and Gleason scores of 8–10 were significant predictors of prostate-cancer-specific mortality after either radical prostatectomy or radiation therapy, as shown in a study comprising over 1000 men.[11]

Prostate size and risk of high-grade, advanced disease and PSA progression after radical prostatectomy. In 1602 men who underwent radical prostatectomy, the smaller the prostate, the higher the proportion of high-grade disease, positive surgical margins, extracapsular extension and biochemical progression. These data suggest that prostate size after surgery should be evaluated as a prognostic factor. They also suggest that for a defined equivalent PSA level in 2 men (e.g. 5 ng/mL), tumor volume is probably very different depending on whether the prostate is large or small. For smaller prostates, the amount of serum PSA cannot be explained by what is produced by the transition zone and most likely the tumor volume accounts for the observed circulating PSA.

These data provide further evidence of the usefulness of PSA volume-derived parameters such as the PSA density of the transition zone for prostate cancer staging.[12]

Other markers

Aberrant promoter hypermethylation. There is an obvious need to find other markers for prostate cancer detection. Aberrant promoter hypermethylation of several tumor suppressor genes occurs frequently during pathogenesis of prostate cancer and is a potential marker for detection of prostate cancer. A test based on a quantitative methylation-specific polymerase chain reaction (PCR) of multiple genes in DNA from urine sediment has been developed and evaluated. Samples from 52 men with prostate cancer and 91 age-matched controls were studied for methylation of nine gene promoters. Overall, the methylation found in urine samples matched the methylation status in primary tumors. With 100% specificity, the sensitivity of a combination of four genes was sufficient to detect only 87% of prostate cancers.[13]

Diagnostic and prognostic information from hypermethylated genes. Promoter CpG island hypermethylation has been hypothesized to play a role in the aggressiveness of prostate cancer. This promoter hypermethylation concept has been investigated as a diagnostic and prognostic tool in prostate cancer. Hypermethylation was highly prevalent at three well-known gene loci (*GSTP1*, *APC* and *PTGS1*), with a sensitivity in the 70–95% range and a specificity above 90%. In addition, the methylation of two or three gene loci correlated with well-known prognostic factors.[14]

In another study looking at the risk of early PSA recurrence following radical prostatectomy in 85 men, the presence of serum DNA with *GSTP1* CpG island hypermethylation was the most significant predictor of PSA recurrence.[15]

Antibody signatures. A new test that looks for antibodies to a panel of 22 antigens derived from prostate cancer tissue could be of major interest in discriminating between patients with prostate cancer and controls. In 60 patients and 68 controls, this 22-biomarker assay achieved a sensitivity of 81.6% and a specificity of 88.2%.[16]

It remains to be seen whether this new antibody signature test can distinguish between indolent and aggressive tumors.

Telomerase activity. Exfoliated cells in the urine are increasingly being studied for their potential use in diagnosis of prostate cancer. In 56 men with proven prostate cancer, telomerase activity assessed by quantitative real-time PCR reached a 100% sensitivity. By contrast, no telomerase activity at all was detected in 70% of patients with benign prostatic hyperplasia (BPH), and only very low levels in another 18%. In the 12% of BPH patients with high levels of telomerase activity, undiagnosed prostate cancer is a possible cause.[17]

Although the series was limited, a 100% sensitivity with a 70%-plus specificity clearly outperforms any other diagnostic test for prostate cancer and this avenue is certainly worth investigating.

Radical prostatectomy versus watchful waiting

In 2002 the initial results of a landmark trial comparing radical prostatectomy with watchful waiting in the management of early prostate cancer were reported. The estimated 10-year results are now available. A total of 347 patients were randomized to radical prostatectomy and 348 to watchful waiting. Median follow-up was

8.2 years. In the radical prostatectomy group, 83 patients died, as did 106 in the watchful-waiting group ($p = 0.04$). There was a 26% reduction in overall mortality, 44% reduction in prostate cancer mortality, 40% reduction in risk of metastases and a 67% reduction in local progression in the radical prostatectomy group. Radical prostatectomy therefore reduces disease-specific and overall mortality, and the risks of metastasis and local progression.[18]

It is worth noting that, when the patients were stratified according to age (65 years and younger; over 65 years), benefits from surgery in patients over 65 years of age were minimal, although the study was not powered to detect this.

Laparoscopic radical prostatectomy

Rassweiler and colleagues analyzed the outcomes of a multicenter study with more than 5500 patients and 50 surgeons in 18 centers in Germany, Austria and Switzerland.[19] The study is strong in terms of patient numbers, but shows weakness in terms of data uniformity. Data are presented in Table 1. The authors concluded that laparoscopic radical prostatectomy has become a safe and effective treatment. There is effective transfer of a difficult technique and the learning curve nowadays is shorter than that for pioneers.

TABLE 1

Laparoscopic radical prostatectomy – findings of a multicenter study[19]

Criteria	Mean	Range
Operating time (min)	196	150–292
Conversion rate (%)	2.4	0–14
Reintervention rate (%)	2.6	0.3–7
Complication rate (%)	8.9	1.8–10.8
Positive margins pT2 tumors (%)	10.6	3.2–18
Continence – 12 months (%)	85	72–94
Potency – 12 months (%)	52.5	35–67
PSA recurrence – pT2 (%)	8.6	4–15

Identifying patients at risk for significant versus clinically insignificant postoperative PSA failure

In 1011 men treated with radical prostatectomy, a preoperative PSA velocity above 2 ng/mL/year and Gleason score above 7 were significantly associated with a postoperative PSA doubling time of less than 3 months. By contrast, select men with intermediate-risk disease and a postoperative doubling time of more than 12 months may not require additional therapy.[20]

20-year outcomes following conservative management of clinically localized prostate cancer

With a median observation of 24 years, a retrospective population-based cohort study looked at 767 men aged 55–74 years with clinically localized prostate cancer diagnosed between 1971 and 1984 (thus representing a quite different patient population from nowadays), who were treated with observation or immediate or delayed androgen withdrawal therapy. The study analyzed the probability of mortality from prostate cancer or other competing medical conditions, given a patient's age at diagnosis and tumor grade. Men with low-grade prostate cancers had a minimal risk of dying from prostate cancer during 20 years of follow-up (Gleason score 2–4; 6 deaths per 1000 person-years). Men with high-grade prostate cancers had a high probability of dying from prostate cancer within 10 years of diagnosis (Gleason score 8–10; 121 deaths per 1000 person-years). Men with a Gleason score of 5 or 6 had an intermediate risk of death from prostate cancer. The annual mortality from prostate cancer appears to remain stable after 15 years from diagnosis, which does not support aggressive treatment for localized low-grade prostate cancer.[21]

Long-term survival rates of patients with prostate cancer in the screening era

Absolute and relative survival rates for 2000 were derived from the 1973–2000 database of the Surveillance, Epidemiology and End Results (SEER) program. Overall, 5- and 10-year relative survival rates were approximately 99% and 95%; that is, excess mortality compared with the general population was as low as 1% and 5% within 5 and 10 years following diagnosis, respectively. Two-thirds of patients were diagnosed with well- or moderately differentiated localized/regional prostate cancer; among these patients, 5- and 10-year relative survival rates were above 100% (indicating the lack of any excess mortality) at all ages.[22] The majority of patients diagnosed with prostate cancer in the PSA screening era do not have excess mortality compared with the general population under current patterns of medical care.

Radiotherapy

High-dose versus conventional-dose radiotherapy. It has often been assumed that the higher the overall dose of radiation, the better the outcome, but this had not been proved by randomized trials. Such a trial was performed in 393 men with T1b–T2b disease and PSA levels below 15 ng/mL. Mean follow-up was 5.5 years. The conventional radiation dose was 70.2 Gy and the high dose 79.2 Gy. The proportion of men free from biochemical failure (i.e. increasing PSA level) at 5 years was 20% higher in the high-dose arm (80.4% vs 61.4%) – a 49% reduction in the risk of biochemical failure. Both low- and high-risk subgroups benefited from high-dose treatment. Major grade-3 or greater morbidity was encountered in a fairly similar proportion (1% for low-dose, 2% for high-dose radiation therapy).[23]

Similarly, the optimal radiation dose in a fractionation schedule was evaluated in a randomized trial of 936 men with T1–T2 disease (66 Gy in 33 fractions over 45 days compared with 52.5 Gy in 20 fractions over 28 days). A slight advantage of 7% was observed in favor of the long-schedule arm, which also had a lower acute toxicity profile; late toxicity was similarly low in both arms (3.2%).[24]

Risk-adapted androgen deprivation combined with high-dose conformal radiotherapy. An interesting, although not randomized, study allocated low-risk patients to three-dimensional conformal therapy alone (n = 181), intermediate-risk patients to 4–6 months' neoadjuvant hormonal therapy prior to radiation treatment (n = 75) and high-risk patients to neoadjuvant and 2 years' adjuvant androgen deprivation following radiotherapy (n = 160).[25]

At 3 years' follow-up (which might be considered too short given the 2-year hormonal therapy in one of the arms), 5-year biochemical disease-free survival lay in the same range for all groups (80, 73 and 79% for low-, intermediate- and high-risk patients, respectively) whereas in most other studies using radiation therapy these figures would have been significantly different for low- and high-risk patients. In agreement with the aforementioned studies, there was also a 20% difference in outcome in favor of high-dose ($\geq$ 72 Gy) over low-dose (< 72 Gy) radiotherapy.

Value of postoperative radiotherapy after radical prostatectomy: an answer at last? The real benefits of radiation therapy after radical prostatectomy have so far been ill-defined. A randomized trial by the European Organization for the Research and Treatment of Cancer (EORTC) compared radical prostatectomy followed by immediate radiotherapy with prostatectomy alone in 1005 patients with pT3 cancer or pT2 cancer with positive margins. After a median follow-up of 5 years, biochemical and clinical progression-free survival was significantly improved in the irradiated group. Whether this will translate later on into an overall survival advantage remains to be proven. Interestingly, even in the subgroup of patients with seminal invasion, radiotherapy had a positive impact on outcome.[26]

Hormonal therapy

Early versus delayed hormonal therapy. Another landmark study from the EORTC, the EORTC 30891 study group, analyzed the advantage of early compared with delayed hormonal therapy in asymptomatic patients with prostate cancer not suitable for definitive local treatment, who were randomized to immediate or delayed endocrine treatments. Results showed no significant differences in PSA survival or overall symptom-free survival. The deferred approach could spare treatment to a substantial number of patients (around 25% in this trial).[27]

Risk of fracture after androgen deprivation for prostate cancer.
The use of androgen-deprivation therapy for prostate cancer is associated with a loss of bone mineral density; however, the risk of fracture after androgen-deprivation therapy has not been studied extensively. The records of 50 613 men who were listed in the databases of the SEER program and Medicare were analyzed. Of men surviving at least 5 years after diagnosis, 19.4% of those who received androgen-deprivation therapy suffered a fracture, compared with 12.6% of those who did not receive the treatment ($p < 0.001$). Thus, androgen-deprivation therapy for prostate cancer increases the risk of fracture.[28]

Structural basis for resistance to bicalutamide in prostate cancer.
Despite androgen-deprivation therapy, prostate cancers often become refractory, as evidenced by PSA values and clinical progression. The key to this resistance may lie in the expression of the androgen receptor itself or its induced modifications. Withdrawal of the anti-androgen results in the regression of PSA in about one-third of cases. Mutation of the bicalutamide receptor may result in bicalutamide having agonistic activity rather than anti-androgen activity, and thus being likely to be involved in the anti-androgen withdrawal syndrome. Knowledge of the binding mechanism for some anti-androgens may explain the stimulatory properties of some of these compounds and provide a molecular rationale for the development of new anti-androgens and selective androgen-receptor modulators.[29]

Natural history of rising serum PSA in men with castrate non-metastatic prostate cancer

An interesting study has described the natural history of non-metastatic prostate cancer and rising PSA despite androgen-deprivation therapy. A total of 201 men were included in the placebo control group from a randomized controlled trial to evaluate the effects of zoledronic acid on time to first bone metastasis in men with prostate cancer, no bone metastases and rising PSA despite androgen-deprivation therapy. At 2 years, 33% of patients had developed bone metastases. Median bone-metastasis-free survival was 30 months. Baseline PSA level above 10 ng/mL and PSA velocity independently predicted shorter time to first bone metastasis. In men with non-metastatic prostate cancer and rising PSA despite androgen-deprivation therapy, the disease has a relatively indolent natural history.[30]

Lack of effect of epidermal growth factor inhibitor on hormone-refractory prostate cancer

A multicenter, randomized, phase II study was undertaken by the National Cancer Institute of Canada Clinical Trials Group to evaluate the efficacy and toxicity of oral gefitinib, an epidermal growth factor inhibitor, in 40 patients with minimally symptomatic, hormone-refractory prostate cancer. Gefitinib did not result in any responses in PSA or objective measurable disease at either dose.[31] These data show that, although now well-known pathways were targeted, men are not big mice and, unfortunately, data from the laboratory cannot always be translated to humans.

Chemotherapy

Early chemotherapy. Usually indicated for metastatic hormone-refractory prostate cancer, several ongoing studies are analyzing the effects of chemotherapy, particularly taxanes, in earlier stages of the disease. In high-risk localized prostate cancer with biopsy Gleason scores between 8 and 10, serum PSA above 20 ng/mL and/or clinical T3 cancer, weekly neoadjuvant docetaxel was given for 6 months to 19 patients. PSA decreases of more than 50% were observed in 11 out of 19 patients (58%), whereas decline in tumor volume of more than 25% (assessed by endorectal magnetic resonance imaging) was confirmed in 68% of them. Sixteen patients completed chemotherapy and underwent radical prostatectomy. Interestingly, none of them achieved complete pathological response.[32]

Highlights in **prostate cancer** *2005–06*

WHAT'S IN?

Diagnosis and monitoring

- Testosterone levels and prostate cancer
- PSA kinetics (PSA velocity before radical prostatectomy or radiotherapy)

Treatment

- Radical prostatectomy (open and laparoscopic) confirmed as an effective treatment for intermediate- and high-risk tumor patients with a life expectancy of more than 10 years
- Conservative management of low-risk prostate cancer in older patients
- High-dose conformal radiotherapy
- Risk-adapted androgen deprivation and radiotherapy
- Immediate postoperative radiotherapy after radical prostatectomy for positive margins
- PSA doubling time for discriminating between significant and insignificant PSA failure after radical prostatectomy
- Simultaneous hormonal therapy and chemotherapy

WHAT'S OUT?

Diagnosis

- 'Static' PSA for diagnosis of early prostate cancer
- Yearly PSA testing if PSA is below 1 ng/mL after the age of 60 years

Treatment

- Bicalutamide monotherapy for localized prostate cancer
- Maximal androgen blockade
- Epidermal growth factor therapy

Highlights in **prostate cancer** 2005–06

WHAT'S NEW?

Diagnosis

- Autoantibody signatures
- Aberrant promoter hypermethylation for diagnosis and prognosis of prostate cancer
- Telomerase activity

Prognosis

- Obesity and biochemical failure

Treatment

- Targeted therapeutic intervention on differentiated androgen-dependent and -independent genes

WHAT'S CONTROVERSIAL?

Diagnosis

- Screening for prostate cancer

Treatment

- Chemotherapy earlier in the disease course
- Early versus late hormonal therapy

Combining hormonal therapy with chemotherapy: timing is of utmost importance. Combining androgen ablation with chemotherapy is a logical idea, but the optimal timing of the two elements is far from established. In the well-known Shionogi and LNCaP xenograft models in mice, simultaneous androgen deprivation and taxane-based chemotherapy was more effective than sequential treatments.[33]

References

1. Lonn E, Bosch J, Yusuf S et al.; HOPE and HOPE-TOO trial investigators. Effects of long-term vitamin E supplementation on cardiovascular events and cancer: a randomized controlled trial. *JAMA* 2005;293:1338–47.

2. Tammela TL, Maattanen L, Martikainen P et al. Preliminary results from the third round of the Finnish prostate cancer screening trial. *Eur Urol Suppl* 2005; 4(3):A596.

3. Aus G, Damber JE, Khatami A et al. PSA and future risk of prostate cancer. *Eur Urol Suppl* 2005;4(3): A123.

4. Roobol MJ, Roobol DW, Schroder FH. Is additional testing necessary in men with prostate-specific antigen levels of 1.0 ng/mL or less in a population-based screening setting? (ERSSPC, section Rotterdam). *Urology* 2005;65:343–6.

5. Baillargeon J, Pollock BH, Kristal AR et al. The association of body mass index and prostate-specific antigen in a population-based study. *Cancer* 2005;103:1092–5.

6. Freedland SJ, Isaacs WB, Mangold LA et al. Stronger association between obesity and biochemical progression after radical prostatectomy among men treated in the last 10 years. *Clin Cancer Res* 2005;11:2883–8.

7. Thompson IM, Ankerst DP, Chi C et al. Operating characteristics of prostate-specific antigen in men with an initial PSA level of 3.0 ng/ml or lower. *JAMA* 2005;294:66–70.

8. Patel DA, Presti JC Jr, McNeal JE et al. Preoperative PSA velocity is an independent prognostic factor for relapse after radical prostatectomy. *J Clin Oncol* 2005;23:6157–62.

9. D'Amico AV, Renshaw AA, Sussman B, Chen MH. Pretreatment PSA velocity and risk of death from prostate cancer following external beam radiation therapy. *JAMA* 2005;294:440–7.

10. Freedland SJ, Humphreys EB, Mangold LA et al. Risk of prostate cancer-specific mortality following biochemical recurrence after radical prostatectomy. *JAMA* 2005;294: 433–9.

11. Zhou P, Chen MH, McLeod D et al. Predictors of prostate cancer-specific mortality after radical prostatectomy or radiation therapy. *J Clin Oncol* 2005;23:6992–8.

12. Freedland SJ, Isaacs WB, Platz EA et al. Prostate size and risk of high-grade, advanced prostate cancer and biochemical progression after radical prostatectomy: a search database study. *J Clin Oncol* 2005;23: 7546–54.

13. Hoque MO, Topaloglu O, Begum S et al. Quantitative methylation-specific polymerase chain reaction gene patterns in urine sediment distinguish prostate cancer patients from control subjects. *J Clin Oncol* 2005;23:6569–75.

14. Bastian PJ, Ellinger J, Wellmann A et al. Diagnostic and prognostic information in prostate cancer with the help of a small set of hypermethylated gene loci. *Clin Cancer Res* 2005;11:4097–106.

15. Bastian PJ, Palapattu GS, Lin X et al. Preoperative serum DNA *GSTP1* CpG island hypermethylation and the risk of early prostate-specific antigen recurrence following radical prostatectomy. *Clin Cancer Res* 2005;11:4037–43.

16. Wang X, Yu J, Sreekumar A et al. Autoantibody signatures in prostate cancer. *N Engl J Med* 2005;353:1224–35.

17. Botchkina GI, Kim RH, Botchkina IL et al. Noninvasive detection of prostate cancer by quantitative analysis of telomerase activity. *Clin Cancer Res* 2005;11:3243–9.

18. Bill-Axelson A, Holmberg L, Ruutu M et al; Scandinavian Prostate Cancer Group Study No. 4. Radical prostatectomy versus watchful waiting in early prostate cancer. *N Engl J Med* 2005;352:1977–84.

19. Rassweiler J, Stolzenburg J, Sulser T et al. Laparoscopic radical prostatectomy – a multi-institutional study with more than 5500 patients. *Eur Urol Suppl* 2005;4(3):A444.

20. D'Amico AV, Chen MH, Roehl KA, Catalona WJ. Identifying patients at risk for significant versus clinically insignificant postoperative prostate-specific antigen failure. *J Clin Oncol* 2005;23:4975–9.

21. Albertsen PC, Hanley JA, Fine J. 20-year outcomes following conservative management of clinically localized prostate cancer. *JAMA* 2005;293:2095–101.

22. Brenner H, Arndt V. Long-term survival rates of patients with prostate cancer in the prostate-specific antigen screening era: population-based estimates for the year 2000 by period analysis. *J Clin Oncol* 2005;23:441–7.

23. Zietman AL, DeSilvio ML, Slater JD et al. Comparison of conventional-dose vs high-dose conformal radiation therapy in clinically localized adenocarcinoma of the prostate: a randomized controlled trial. *JAMA* 2005;294:1233–9.

24. Lukka H, Hayter C, Julian JA et al. Randomized trial comparing two fractionation schedules for patients with localized prostate cancer. *J Clin Oncol* 2005;23:6132–8.

25. Zapatero A, Valcarcel F, Calvo FA et al. Risk-adapted androgen deprivation and escalated three-dimensional conformal radiotherapy for prostate cancer: Does radiation dose influence outcome of patients treated with adjuvant androgen deprivation? A GICOR study. *J Clin Oncol* 2005;23:6561–8.

26. Bolla M, van Poppel H, Collette L et al; European Organization for Research and Treatment of Cancer. Postoperative radiotherapy after radical prostatectomy: a randomised controlled trial (EORTC trial 22911). *Lancet* 2005;366:572–8.

27. Studer UE, Whelan P, Albrecht W et al. Patients with asymptomatic prostate cancer T0–4 N0–2 M0 not suitable for local definitive treatment: do they need immediate androgen deprivation? *Eur Urol Suppl* 2005; 4(3):A303.

28. Shahinian VB, Kuo YF, Freeman JL, Goodwin JS. Risk of fracture after androgen deprivation for prostate cancer. *N Engl J Med* 2005;352:154–64.

29. Bohl CE, Gao W, Miller DD et al. Structural basis for antagonism and resistance of bicalutamide in prostate cancer. *Proc Natl Acad Sci USA* 2005;102:6201–6.

30. Smith MR, Kabbinavar F, Saad F et al. Natural history of rising serum prostate-specific antigen in men with castrate nonmetastatic prostate cancer. *J Clin Oncol* 2005;23: 2918–25.

31. Canil CM, Moore MJ, Winquist E et al. Randomized phase II study of two doses of gefitinib in hormone-refractory prostate cancer: a trial of the National Cancer Institute of Canada Clinical Trials Group. *J Clin Oncol* 2005;23:455–60.

32. Febbo PG, Richie JP, George DJ et al. Neoadjuvant docetaxel before radical prostatectomy in patients with high-risk localized prostate cancer. *Clin Cancer Res* 2005;11:5233–40.

33. Eigl BJ, Eggener SE, Baybik J et al. Timing is everything: preclinical evidence supporting simultaneous rather than sequential chemo-hormonal therapy for prostate cancer. *Clin Cancer Res* 2005;11:4905–11.

Bladder tumors

Mark S Soloway MD

Department of Urology, University of Miami School of Medicine, Miami, Florida, USA

Bladder tumors are one of the common neoplasms in many areas throughout the world. Although cigarette smoking is likely one factor, there are probably many environmental carcinogens that are responsible. There may also be host factors that will become evident once there is a better understanding of the molecular events involved with carcinogenesis. For example, I was recently told that despite a relatively high prevalence of bladder tumors in Turkey, in part related to cigarette smoking, the vast majority are confined to the urothelium and are low grade.

Management of papillary tumors

Many papillary tumors of the bladder act in a benign manner and, according to the 2004 World Health Organization/International Society of Urological Pathology classification, are termed papilloma, papillary neoplasm of low malignant potential, and low-grade non-invasive (Ta) tumors.[1] It is incumbent on the urologist to remove these tumors to establish a diagnosis and then to monitor and treat the patient with the primary goal of preserving normal bladder function, avoiding overtreatment and preventing tumor growth to the extent that bleeding results. In the vast majority of patients, this can be initially accomplished with a thorough endoscopic resection followed by a single dose of intravesical chemotherapy. If the first 3-month cystoscopy is negative, some guidelines indicate the next endoscopy can be 9 months later.[2,3] As long as there is no high-grade urothelial tumor, there is no urgency to detect a subsequent tumor. If there is concern about waiting 9 months, urine can be analyzed by cytology or a sensitive tumor marker. If either is positive, cystoscopy can be performed. Many subsequent low-grade papillary tumors are small and easily treated with office fulguration or monitored until they require removal.[4] BCG (bacillus Calmette–Guérin) is not indicated for low-grade Ta tumors as the risks outweigh the potential benefit.[2,3]

Intravesical gemcitabine has been introduced as a new treatment for Ta tumors, with some efficacy.[5] Its role has yet to be defined, as the number of patients treated to date has been few. It has been well tolerated.

Adjuvant intravesical chemotherapy

Several years ago I polled 500 clinicians at the annual meeting of the American Urological Association. Only 10% routinely gave intravesical chemotherapy immediately after transurethral resection (TUR). More recent informal polls suggest the vast majority either give it or believe it is appropriate and are trying to navigate the local hospital and nursing regulations that make instillation of chemotherapy in the recovery room difficult. Several well-performed randomized trials (RCTs) have established the benefit of this approach in reducing the risk of a subsequent tumor, presumably by lessening the chance of tumor implantation.[6–8] One important contraindication to postoperative chemotherapy is bladder perforation. Extravasation of mitomycin or epirubicin results in an intense inflammatory reaction and must be avoided. Parenthetically, BCG can also produce a most undesirable perivesical inflammatory reaction if it extravasates.[9]

Upper-tract monitoring

The risk of an upper-tract tumor in an individual with one or more low-grade Ta tumors is very low, and routine monitoring of the upper urinary tract (UUT) is not recommended.[2,3] In general, surveillance of the UUT in patients with bladder cancer has not been shown to be effective in reducing death from an UUT tumor. Although the risk of an upper-tract tumor may approach 15–20% over 15 years in some subgroups (i.e. carcinoma in situ, CIS), the interval between radiographs is usually 6 months to 2 years, and the great majority of patients who develop a life-threatening (high-grade) UUT tumor present with hematuria or pain between such monitoring studies. More frequent monitoring with cytology or a tumor marker would seem to be more productive. A positive result will, of course, not reveal the location of neoplastic cells; however, if the lower tract is normal, the UUT should be investigated.

The approach to patients with high-grade Ta and T1 urothelial cancer of the bladder has undergone a subtle but very important change over the last couple of years. Accurate staging and complete resection is critical. Since understaging can delay a recommendation to proceed with a radical cystectomy (RC) and the results with BCG are better if the patient starts with a complete resection, the current guideline is to return the patient to the operating room for a second TUR within a month after a transurethral resection of a T1 tumor.[10,11] Many advocate the same for any high-grade Ta tumor. Several studies report understaging 25% of patients with the initial TUR. Not surprisingly, the 'reTUR' results in a change in therapy in some patients and avoids a 3-month delay in proceeding with a RC if the reTUR reveals a T2 lesion. If the second TUR reveals high-grade Ta or T1 (or T0), then a 6-week course of BCG is generally recommended, unless RC is still felt to be the best choice. Any high-grade recurrence or new tumor at 3 months is an indication for RC. If there is no tumor at 3 months, maintenance BCG for at least 1 year reduces the recurrence rate.[12] Side effects due to BCG can often be managed by reducing the dose of BCG by two-thirds.[13,14] It is imperative, however, not to allow undue delay in proceeding with a RC if there is high-grade urothelial cancer not readily accessible to complete endoscopic excision.

The term 'superficial' bladder cancer should be avoided since, as it is currently used, it includes Ta, T1 and CIS. It has traditionally been used to designate any tumor that can be removed by endoscopic resection. Unfortunately, it implies a relatively good prognosis – note 'superficial' and, therefore, not 'deep'. This is not uniformly correct, of course. A low-grade Ta tumor has a very different prognosis from a high-grade T1. Most importantly, by definition the word 'superficial' means 'lying on'. A T1 tumor is not confined to the surface and should not be called a superficial bladder tumor.[15]

Muscle invasion

Once a bladder tumor invades the muscle, the risk of metastasis rises substantially. Randomized trials have explored the use of systemic chemotherapy both as induction (pre-RC) and as adjuvant (post-RC) treatment.[16–18] The trials included patients with cT2 and T3. There is an approximate 5% survival benefit with neoadjuvant methotrexate–vinblastine–doxorubicin–cisplatin (MVAC). If all patients with cT2 receive neoadjuvant chemotherapy, many patients will receive chemotherapy without benefit either because they are cured by RC alone or because they do not respond, meaning that surgery is delayed while response is sought. Some 30% of patients receiving neoadjuvant chemotherapy are pT0 after RC (compared with 10% without preoperative chemotherapy), indicating that MVAC is active in this setting. It is my practice to begin with chemotherapy in patients with cT3 or with hydronephrosis (if the renal function is satisfactory).

Lymphovascular invasion

Lymphovascular invasion associated with urothelial carcinoma of the bladder is an adverse prognostic factor. When the pathologist conveys its presence in a T1 lesion, it should prompt either an aggressive reTUR or cystectomy. If observed in the TUR specimen of a cT2–T3 lesion, it might suggest induction chemotherapy; and if noted following a cystectomy, it may prompt adjuvant systemic chemotherapy. I am not aware of any RCTs that support this approach; however, the adverse implication of small vessel invasion is consistent among many reports.

The chemotherapeutic regimen of gemcitabine–cisplatin is less toxic than MVAC but has not been tested in the neoadjuvant setting. It is not a huge leap of faith to substitute it if the oncologist feels more comfortable thus.

An alternative approach is to proceed with a RC and make a decision regarding chemotherapy after the RC. This provides the benefit of pathological staging. One disadvantage is that any postoperative complications may delay initiation of chemotherapy, and up to 25% of patients have some complications after a RC.

Some patients refuse chemotherapy after having undergone this major surgery ('physician fatigue').

There may be several treatment options for the following clinical scenarios:

- clinical T2–T3b transitional cell carcinoma
- transitional cell carcinoma of the prostatic ducts or stroma
- high-grade T1 or CIS after failure with BCG
- multifocal T1 plus CIS.

However, RC remains the preferred approach to which other avenues must be compared. Bladder preservation with a 'complete' TUR with or without cisplatin combination chemotherapy and with or without radiation may provide similar disease-specific survival in highly selected patients.[19] The optimal candidate for bladder preservation is someone with a small cT2 tumor without CIS and following a complete TUR and probably a reTUR to confirm the absence of residual tumor in the muscle. There should be no hydronephrosis. The patient must be committed to life-long surveillance. Fewer than one-third of my patients fulfill these criteria.

Is cystectomy being denied?

A recent report indicated that in many parts of the USA fewer than 50% of patients who have muscle-invasive bladder cancer undergo a RC.[20] This is particularly true if the patients are over 75 years old. There is a perception that RC is a very high-risk procedure and that patients older than 75 are unfit for it, but many reports indicate this to be incorrect.[21,22] The perioperative mortality is less than 3% across all age groups, and age alone is not a contraindication to RC. Although surgery is indeed best performed in centers with sufficient experience, patients may not be willing to travel for their care.

New techniques have improved radical cystectomy, notably by reducing operative time and blood loss. The automatic stapling device, the LigaSure (Valleylab, Boulder, CO, USA) and the harmonic scalpel have all contributed toward this. Some skilled surgeons have successfully performed laparoscopic RC, usually with

Highlights in **bladder tumors** *2005–06*

WHAT'S IN?

- Chip camera built into flexible cystoscope
- Continuous flow resection
- Second transurethral resection (TUR) for high grade Ta-T1
- Intravesical chemotherapy after transurethral resection of a bladder tumor
- Maintenance BCG (bacillus Calmette–Guérin)
- Prostate sparing for very select patients
- Staging prostatic urethral transitional cell carcinoma
- Neoadjuvant chemotherapy for cT3
- Gemcitabine–cisplatin
- Selective monitoring of upper tract depending on risk category

WHAT'S OUT?

- The term 'superficial bladder cancer'
- Looking through the lens
- Bladder perforation during TUR
- Upper urinary tract monitoring for Ta
- Neoadjuvant treatment for cT2

a small incision to perform the diversion. I do not envision a rapid transition to this approach.

The first International Consultation on Bladder Tumors was held in Hawaii, October 3–7, 2004. Experts from around the globe contributed to the development of guidelines for the diagnosis and treatment of this disease. A text that details the report has just become available.

References

1. Epstein JI, Amin MB, Ruter VR, Mostafi FK. The World Health Organization/International Society of Urological Pathology Consensus Classification of Urothelial (transitional cell) Neoplasms of the Urinary Bladder. Bladder Consensus Conference Committee. *Am J Surg Pathol* 1998;22:1435–48.

2. Oosterlinck W, Lobel B, Jakse G et al.; EAU Working Group on Oncological Urology. Guidelines on Bladder Cancer. *Eur Urol* 2002;41:105–12.

3. Oosterlinck W, Solsona E, Akaza H et al. Low-grade Ta (non-invasive) urothelial carcinoma of the bladder. *Urology* 2005; 66(6 suppl 1):75–89.

4. Soloway MS, Bruck DS, Kim SS. Expectant management of small, recurrent, non-invasive papillary bladder tumors. *J Urol* 2003; 170:438–41.

5. Dalbagni G, Russo P, Sheinfeld J et al. Phase I trial of intravesical gemcitabine in bacillus Calmette–Guérin refractory transitional cell carcinoma of the bladder. *J Clin Oncol* 2002;20:3193–8.

6. Weldon T, Soloway M. Susceptibility of urothelium to neoplastic cellular implantation. *Urology* 1975;5:824–7.

7. Soloway M, Masters S. Urothelial susceptibility to tumor cell implantation, influence of cauterization. *Cancer* 1980;46:1158–63.

8. Sylvester R, Oosterlinck W, van der Meijden A. A single, immediate post-operative instillation of chemotherapy decreases the risk of recurrence in patients with stage Ta, T1 bladder cancer: a meta-analysis of published results of randomized clinical trials. *J Urol* 2004;171:2181–5.

9. Nieder AM, Sved PD, Stein JP et al. Cystoprostatectomy and orthotopic ileal neobladder reconstruction for management of bacille Calmette–Guérin-induced bladder contractures. *Urology* 2005;65:909–12.

10. Sylvester RJ, van der Meijden A, Witjes JA et al. High-grade urothelial carcinoma and carcinoma in situ of the bladder. *Urology* 2005;66 (6 suppl 1):90–107.

11. Nieder AM, Brausi M, Lamm D et al. Management of stage T1 tumors of the bladder: International Consensus Panel. *Urology* 2005;66 (6 suppl 1):108–25.

12. Lamm DL, Blumenstein BA, Crissman JD et al. Maintenance bacillus Calmette–Guérin immunotherapy for recurrent Ta, T1 and carcinoma in situ transitional cell carcinoma of the bladder: a randomized Southwest Oncology Group Study. *J Urol* 2000;163: 1124–9.

13. Martinez-Pinero JA, Flores N, Isorna S et al. Long term follow-up of a randomized prospective trial comparing a standard 81 mg dose of intravesical bacillus Calmette–Guérin with a reduced dose of 27 mg in superficial bladder cancer. *BJU Int* 2002;89:671–80.

14. Losa A, Hurley R, Lembo A. Low dose bacillus Calmette–Guérin for carcinoma in situ of the bladder: long term results. *J Urol* 2000;163:68–72.

15. Nieder AM, Soloway MS. Eliminate the term "superficial" bladder cancer. *J Urol* 2006;175: 417–18.

16. Grossman HB, Natale RB, Tangen CM et al. Neoadjuvant chemotherapy plus cystectomy compared with cystectomy alone for locally advanced bladder cancer. *N Engl J Med* 2003;349:859–66.

17. Sternberg C, Donat SM, Ballmunt J et al. Chemotherapy for bladder cancer: treatment guidelines for neoadjuvant chemotherapy, bladder preservation, adjuvant chemotherapy and metastatic cancer. *Urology* 2006; in press.

18. Advanced Bladder Cancer: A Meta-analysis Collaboration. Neoadjuvant chemotherapy in invasive bladder cancer: a systematic review and meta-analysis. *Lancet* 2003;361:1927–34.

19. Shipley W, Kaufman D, Zehr E et al. Selective bladder preservation by combined modality protocol treatment: long-term outcomes of 190 patients with invasive bladder cancer. *Urology* 2002;60:62–7.

20. Prout GR Jr, Wesley MN, Yancik R et al. Age and comorbidity impact surgical therapy in older bladder carcinoma patients: a population-based study: *Cancer* 2005;104:1638–47.

21. Stein JP, Lieskovsky G, Cote R et al. Radical cystectomy in the treatment of invasive bladder cancer. Long-term results in 1,054 patients. *J Clin Oncol* 2001;19:666–75.

22. Chang SS, Labert SG, Cookson MS, Smith JA Jr. Radical cystectomy is safe in elderly patients at high risk. *J Urol* 2001;166:938–41.

Renal cell carcinoma

David Hrouda* MD FRCS(Urol) and
Timothy J Christmas*† MD FRCS(Urol) FEBU
*Charing Cross Hospital, London, UK; †The Royal Marsden Hospital,
London, UK

Etiology

The etiology of renal cell carcinoma (RCC) remains an enigma.
Research suggests an association between RCC and smoking, obesity
and hypertension, supported by a prospective study in a population
of over 150 000 nurses and health professionals. In multivariate
analysis, higher body mass index was confirmed as a risk factor for
women, smoking was a risk factor for men and women, and a
diagnosis of hypertension was associated with a relative risk of 1.9 in
both men and women.[1] A study from the Netherlands found a non-
significant increase in risk for RCC in patients with a diagnosis of
hypertension, but the association was stronger in patients with RCC
who had somatic von Hippel–Lindau gene mutations.[2]

Tumor staging

It is now accepted that the TNM staging cut-off of 7 cm defined in
1997 to separate T1 from T2 tumors was too high. The *American
Joint Committee on Cancer Staging Manual* (6th edn) now defines:
- T1a tumors as not greater than 4 cm
- T1b tumors as greater than 4 cm but not greater than 7 cm.

However, the debate about which cut-off level is most predictive
of cancer-specific survival continues. Elmore and colleagues have
suggested using a cut-off of 5 cm.[3] A recent European study of
1138 patients had similar findings, with an optimal tumor-size
breakpoint of 5.5 cm.[4]

Roberts et al. reported that 31% of clinical T1 lesions were
pT3a. Interestingly, 5-year recurrence-free survival was the same
for patients upgraded to pT3a and pT1 patients.[5]

The Mayo Clinic group has developed a scoring algorithm to predict survival for patients with metastatic clear-cell RCC.[6] All patients start with a score of 0, and points are added or subtracted for:

- constitutional symptoms at nephrectomy (+2)
- metastases to bone (+2) or liver (+4)
- metastases in multiple sites (+2)
- metastases at nephrectomy (+1) or within 2 years of nephrectomy (+3)
- complete resection of all metastatic sites (−5)
- tumor thrombus level 1–4 (+3)
- primary pathological features of nuclear grade 4 (+3)
- histological tumor necrosis (+2).

Cancer-specific survival rates at 1 year were:

- 85.1% for scores −5 to −1
- 72.1% for scores 0–2
- 58.8% for scores 3–6
- 39.0% for scores 7–8
- 25.1% for scores of 9 and over.

This should prove a useful stratification tool for future trials.

Surgical treatment

Laparoscopic radical nephrectomy. Oncological data that support laparoscopic radical nephrectomy as the gold standard for the management of T1 RCC continue to accrue. The Johns Hopkins group compared outcomes for laparoscopic radical nephrectomy in 73 patients with clinical T1/2 RCC followed for a median 73 months and a similar group of patients undergoing open radical nephrectomy. There was no significant difference in 5- and 10-year disease-specific survival or overall survival.[7] Steinberg and colleagues showed that laparoscopic radical nephrectomy is safe and efficacious in larger tumors (T2); operative time, analgesic requirements, hospital stay, convalescence and complication rates were equivalent to those in patients with tumors of less than 7 cm.[8]

Laparoscopic partial nephrectomy. The Johns Hopkins group reported on the results of laparoscopic partial nephrectomy in

223 patients with a mean tumor size of 2.6 cm.[9] Warm ischemia was employed for 75% of cases, with a mean warm ischemia time of 27.6 minutes. Mean blood loss was 385 mL; the perioperative transfusion rate was 6.9%. Postoperative complications included ileus (1.8%), bleeding (1.8%) and urinary leak (1.4%). The final pathology was RCC in only 66.4% of cases, perhaps reflecting the small mean tumor size. The positive margin rate was 3.5%.

Laparoscopic partial nephrectomy can be performed by either transperitoneal or retroperitoneal routes. Transperitoneal access offers a larger working space and superior instrument angles, and is the better approach for anterior tumors and large or deeply infiltrating posterior tumors. The retroperitoneal approach, although more technically demanding, provides better access for posterior tumors and particularly for posteromedial tumors. In the Cleveland Clinic practice, transperitoneal laparoscopic partial nephrectomy was associated with larger tumors, more calyceal repairs and longer ischemic time, reflected in the slightly longer length of stay (2.9 days compared with 2.2 days for the retroperitoneal approach).[10]

Gill and colleagues demonstrated that, in skilled hands, laparoscopic partial nephrectomy is feasible for hilar tumors.[11] Using en-bloc hilar clamping with cold excision and suture reconstruction in 25 patients, the mean warm ischemia time was 36.4 minutes, with negative margins in all patients, and no kidney was lost for technical reasons.

Laparoscopic partial nephrectomy may also be feasible for selected patients with synchronous ipsilateral renal tumors.[12] The approach included en-bloc partial nephrectomy encompassing both tumors; individual excisions of renal tumors during the same procedure; and partial nephrectomy, with the other tumor treated by cryoablation. All procedures (n = 13) were completed successfully without need for conversion to an open procedure.

Currently, the majority of laparoscopic partial nephrectomies are performed under warm ischemia. However, the true impact of different warm ischemia times on the human kidney is unknown. The Cleveland Clinic group used serum creatinine concentrations to assess renal function before and after laparoscopic partial nephrectomy in patients with a single kidney, and renal scintigraphy in patients with two functioning kidneys.[13] In the latter group, with a warm ischemia time of 30 minutes, function in the kidney that was operated on was reduced by a mean of 29%. In the patients with a single kidney, the mean creatinine concentrations at baseline and at 5-month follow-up were 1.2 and 1.8 mg/dL, respectively. Advancing age and pre-existing azotemia increased the risk of renal dysfunction after laparoscopic partial nephrectomy.

Radiofrequency ablation (RFA). The main argument in favor of energy ablation techniques is the low morbidity compared with open or laparoscopic partial nephrectomy. The majority of reports have focused on radiological criteria of success with relatively short follow-up. The group from Massachusetts General Hospital has reported on the results of treating 100 tumors over a 6-year period.[14] The absence of enhancement on computed tomography or magnetic resonance imaging (MRI) after RFA was interpreted as complete coagulation necrosis. All tumors of less than 3 cm and all exophytic tumors underwent 'complete necrosis' after a single treatment session, but many larger tumors required a second session. Complications were mainly self-limiting or easily treated and included major hemorrhage (2) and ureteral injury (2). The Johns Hopkins group, with 2-year follow-up in 49 patients, found three recurrences at 24–31 months after RFA, all in patients with central tumors larger than 3 cm.[15] In another study, experience with RFA in 60 patients followed up for at least a year showed successful initial ablation in 98% of patients, with one local recurrence that required reablation.[16]

Although these results appear promising for peripheral tumors smaller than 3 cm, many renal masses of this size are indolent. It is therefore likely that 10-year follow-up data will be required to assess the true efficacy of this treatment.

Cryotherapy. Gill and colleagues have published 3-year outcome data on laparoscopic renal cryoablation in 56 patients with a mean

Highlights *in* **renal cell carcinoma** *2005–06*

WHAT'S NEW?

- Raf kinase and VEGF receptor inhibitors for metastatic RCC

WHAT'S IN?

- Laparoscopic radical nephrectomy for T1/T2 RCC
- Laparoscopic partial nephrectomy for T1a RCC

WHAT'S OUT?

- Open radical nephrectomy for T1 RCC

WHAT NEEDS FURTHER EVALUATION?

- Radiofrequency ablation and cryotherapy for small renal masses

tumor size of 2.3 cm.[17] The size of the cryolesion diminished on serial MRI scans over a 3-year period, with 38% of patients having no visible lesion at 3 years. Needle biopsy was performed routinely at 6 months, with findings of persistent tumor in 2 patients. Complications were minimal. As for RFA, long-term survival data are still awaited.

Treatment of metastatic disease

RCC is well known to be resistant to cytotoxic chemotherapy and radiotherapy and has very low complete response rates to interleukin-2 (IL-2). However, there is great optimism about the possible treatment of metastatic disease with a number of novel compounds currently being tested in clinical trials.

Somatic inactivation of the von Hippel–Lindau tumor suppressor gene leads to induction of hypoxia-related genes, including those coding for vascular endothelial growth factor (VEGF) and platelet-derived growth factor (PDGF). Molecular targets for new drugs include interfering with the VEGF receptor or the Raf kinase pathway, inhibition of angiogenesis and antimicrotubule agents. Drugs that interfere with the growth-factor pathways include SU011248, AG-013736, bevacizumab and erlotinib.

The most promising new drug to date is BAY 43-9006 (sorafenib), an oral drug that inhibits tumor-cell proliferation and angiogenesis by inhibition of Raf kinase and VEGF receptors. A phase III study in 769 patients whose RCC had progressed despite treatment with interferon or IL-2 was reported at the American Society of Clinical Oncology (ASCO) meeting in 2005.[18] The drug doubled the time to progression, from 12 weeks to 24 weeks ($p = 0.000001$) with tumor necrosis and shrinkage occurring in the majority of patients. The drug was well tolerated with manageable side effects. Although it is too early to know the impact on overall survival, there is little doubt that this drug has activity against RCC.[18]

References

1. Flaherty KT, Fuchs CS, Colditz GA et al. A prospective study of body mass index, hypertension, and smoking and the risk of renal cell carcinoma (United States). *Cancer Causes Control* 2005;16:1099–106.

2. Schouten LJ, van Dijk BA, Oosterwijk E et al. Hypertension, antihypertensives and mutations in the von Hippel–Lindau gene in renal cell carcinoma: results from the Netherlands Cohort Study. *J Hypertens* 2005;23:1997–2004.

3. Elmore JM, Kadesky KT, Koeneman KS, Sagalowsky AI. Reassessment of the 1997 TNM classification system for renal cell carcinoma. *Cancer* 2003;98:2329–34.

4. Ficarra V, Guille F, Schips L et al. Proposal for revision of the TNM classification system for renal cell carcinoma. *Cancer* 2005;104: 2116–23.

5. Roberts WW, Bhayani SB, Allaf ME et al. Pathological stage does not alter the prognosis for renal lesions determined to be stage T1 by computerized tomography. *J Urol* 2005;173:713–15.

6. Leibovitch BC, Cheville JC, Lohse CM et al. A scoring algorithm to predict survival for patients with metastatic clear cell renal cell carcinoma: a stratification tool for prospective clinical trials. *J Urol* 2005;174:1759–63.

7. Permpongkosol S, Chan DY, Link RE et al. Long-term survival analysis after laparoscopic radical nephrectomy. *J Urol* 2005;174: 1222–5.

8. Steinberg AP, Finelli A, Desai MM et al. Laparoscopic radical nephrectomy for large (greater than 7 cm, T2) renal tumors. *J Urol* 2005;172:2172–6.

9. Link RE, Bhayani SB, Allaf ME et al. Exploring the learning curve, pathological outcomes and perioperative morbidity of laparoscopic partial nephrectomy performed for renal mass. *J Urol* 2005;173:1690–4.

10. Ng CS, Gill IS, Ramani AP et al. Transperitoneal versus retroperitoneal laparoscopic partial nephrectomy: patient selection and perioperative outcomes. *J Urol* 2005;174:846–9.

11. Gill IS, Colombo JR Jr, Frank I et al. Laparoscopic partial nephrectomy for hilar tumors. *J Urol* 2005;174:850–3.

12. Steinberg AP, Kilciler M, Abreu SC et al. Laparoscopic nephron-sparing surgery for two or more ipsilateral renal tumors. *Urology* 2004;64:255–8.

13. Desai MM, Gill IS, Ramani AP et al. The impact of warm ischaemia on renal function after laparoscopic partial nephrectomy. *BJU Int* 2005;95: 377–83.

14. Gervais DA, McGovern FJ, Arellano RS et al. Radiofrequency ablation of renal cell carcinoma: part I. Indications, results, and role in patient management over a 6-year period and ablation of 100 tumors. *Am J Roentgenol* 2005;185:64–71.

15. Varkarakis IM, Allaf ME, Inagaki T et al. Percutaneous radio frequency ablation of renal masses: results at a 2-year mean follow up. *J Urol* 2005;174:456–60.

16. Matsumoto ED, Johnson DB, Ogan K et al. Short-term efficacy of temperature-based radiofrequency ablation of small renal tumors. *Urology* 2005;65:877–81.

17. Gill IS, Remer EM, Hasan WA et al. Renal cryoablation: outcome at 3 years. *J Urol* 2005;173:1903–7.

18. Escudier B, Szczylik C, Eisen T et al. Randomized phase III trial of the Raf kinase and VEGFR inhibitor sorafenib (BAY 43-9006) in patients with advanced renal cell carcinoma (RCC). *Proceedings of American Society of Clinical Oncology Annual Meeting*, Orlando, Florida, USA: 2005; Abstract 4510. www.asco. org/ac/1,1003,_12-002636-00_18-0034-00_19-0032211,00.asp

Laparoscopy, minimally invasive surgery and stone disease

Nicholas Hegarty MD PhD and Inderbir S Gill MD MCh

Section of Laparoscopic and Robotic Surgery, Glickman Urological Institute, Cleveland Clinic Foundation, Cleveland, Ohio, USA

The last year has seen continued growth in the field of minimally invasive urology. New treatment modalities for the treatment of various aspects of urologic disease have been introduced. Imaging and new subtleties of technique have improved on established minimally invasive procedures. At the same time studies with longer-term follow-up have confirmed the safety and efficacy of existing techniques.

Kidney

Laparoscopic nephrectomy has become widely available; currently the majority of urologists in community practice in the USA offer laparoscopy as a treatment option.[1] The 5- and 10-year data that have become available recently suggest that laparoscopic nephrectomy has equivalent outcomes to open nephrectomy for T1 and T2 renal tumors.[2] The increasing number of incidental small tumors that are detected has continued to fuel growth in the field of minimally invasive nephron-sparing surgery. Observational studies have shown that a proportion of these lesions will grow little or not at all if left untreated, and exciting data are emerging using cell biology techniques to predict the behavior of individual incidentalomas.[3] The development of a reliable scheme to detect such indolent tumors will certainly be a great advance, but until then active treatment will be strongly recommended for all surgically fit patients presenting with a renal tumor. Laparoscopic partial nephrectomy (LPN) remains the most widely accepted minimally invasive nephron-sparing technique. With increasing experience, particularly in the last 3–4 years, the complexity of cases being undertaken has expanded considerably. Thus, in specialist centers the indications for LPN currently include select completely intrarenal and central tumors,[4] while laparoscopic heminephrectomy can be performed with surgical outcomes comparable to those for less extensive resections.[5] The duration of warm ischemia time restricts the complexity of surgery, unless cooling is employed. Emerging animal data suggest that warm ischemia times of 90 minutes can be endured with eventual full recovery in solitary kidney models.[6] It is hard to know if such durations will be possible in humans – while renal artery clamping in patients with a solitary kidney can be tolerated for up to 55 minutes, albeit with persisting renal impairment, return of serum creatinine to baseline levels can only be reliably predicted with warm ischemia times of no more than 30 minutes.[7]

Probe ablative therapies provide a means of treating renal tumors without hilar clamping. Following encouraging early results with laparoscopic cryoablation,[8] evolution of technology now allows cryoablation to be performed percutaneously. Preliminary series show satisfactory localization and targeting of the tumor in most cases.[9,10] Oncological outcomes are expected to mirror those of laparoscopic cryoablation; however, given the proximity of overlying structures to the kidney, use is restricted to posterior and posterolateral tumors. Morbidity is low, with studies reporting major complications for cryoablation and radiofrequency ablation (RFA) in 1.8% and minor complications in 9.2% of patients.[11] Early success rates of the order of 98% are reported for RFA.[12] Success is usually defined as absence of enhancement of the ablation site on follow-up radiological imaging. More long-term data are required for the ability of these modalities to induce complete tumor-cell kill to be truly assessed.

Prostate

Use of the da Vinci robot in minimally invasive approaches to prostate cancer has continued its phenomenal growth over the last year. A steep (short) learning curve has been reported for those adept at open surgery,[13] and thus many surgeons have embraced this technology. This in turn has meant that considerably more patients have benefited from minimally invasive surgery. Results that are comparable with those of open surgery are reported in terms of margin status and return of continence. Blood loss and transfusion requirements are consistently lower with laparoscopic and robotic approaches than with open surgery. Robotic-assisted laparoscopic prostatectomy remains 20–30% more expensive than open or laparoscopic prostatectomy,[14] a factor that continues to slow universal acceptance.

Menon and colleagues report retention of potency (defined as the ability to have penetrative intercourse) in up to 97% of men (including those using oral or injection therapies) following robotic-assisted laparoscopic prostatectomy, or in 51% when defined more rigorously as a Sexual Health Inventory for Men (SHIM) score of 21 out of 25 or more.[15] The authors stress that the patients had full potency before surgery.

Another approach that reduces the rate of nerve injury involves imaging with dynamic transrectal ultrasound during surgery. Nerve bundles can be localized on the basis of the flow characteristics of the vascular component of the neurovascular bundles during dissection (Figure 1). Ultrasound also assists identification of the

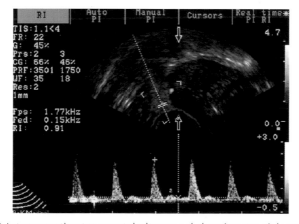

Figure 1 Intraoperative transrectal ultrasound showing arterial waveform in the right neurovascular bundle. (Image courtesy of Dr Osamu Ukimura, Glickman Urological Institute, Cleveland, USA.)

extraprostatic extension of the tumor during surgery and the contour of the apex prior to dissection. Using this technique, a reduction in the rate of positive margins from 21% to 5% in pT2 disease and from 57% to 18% in pT3 has been reported.[16]

A number of other technologies are also being explored, including optical coherence tomography and fluorescence studies. These give details of nerve location and structural integrity, but do not give functional information. Avoidance of thermal energy in the region of the prostate pedicles and the nerve bundles during dissection also aids nerve preservation during laparoscopy.[17] A similar technique has been adopted in robot prostatectomy.[18]

Prostate cryotherapy has an established role as a salvage treatment for recurrence following radiation. Improved technology, including urethral warming, has lessened associated morbidity, and early data for its use as a primary treatment in prostate malignancy are becoming available.[19] It has also been proposed for focal therapy in prostate cancer. Potential problems with this include ruling out other foci of cancer in a disease that is predominantly multifocal, and difficulty in interpreting fluctuations in prostate-specific antigen on follow-up in the presence of retained prostatic tissue.

High-intensity focused ultrasound (HIFU) is re-emerging as a minimally invasive therapy in prostate cancer. It is a bloodless procedure and can be performed in an outpatient setting;[20] however, the brevity of follow-up does not allow conclusions about its efficacy to be drawn. Like cryotherapy, HIFU has been suggested as a treatment modality for focal prostate cancer therapy, but again is subject to the problems of assessing complete tumor eradication.

Bladder

Laparoscopic radical cystectomy series demonstrate the feasibility of performing this surgery.[21] Results in terms of blood loss, morbidity and early oncological outcomes are for the most part encouraging, but longer-term oncological data are awaited.

Highlights in **laparoscopy, minimally invasive surgery and stone disease** *2005–06*

WHAT'S IN?

- Robot-assisted prostatectomy
- Intraoperative imaging during prostatectomy
- Cautery-free nerve dissection
- Percutaneous probe ablation of small renal masses
- Tubeless percutaneous nephrolithotomy

WHAT'S OUT?

- Shock-wave lithotripsy for large stones

WHAT'S ON THE WAY?

- Renal tumor biopsy prognostic molecular markers

Stone disease

The updated American Urological Association guidelines for the treatment of staghorn calculi again support the role of percutaneous surgery for stones greater than 1 cm in diameter.[22] Although tubeless percutaneous nephrolithotomy is not new, having been described in 1984 by Wickham and colleagues,[23] in the last year a number of large series supporting it as a valuable technique have been reported. Blood loss is low, even in bilateral procedures, and hospital stay is reduced without compromising patient safety or outcome.[24]

Regarding the etiology of nephrolithiasis, a number of recent publications have identified obesity as a risk for stone formation.[25] Fortunately, continued scope improvement has allowed a shift away from shock-wave lithotripsy (SWL) towards flexible ureteroscopy for the treatment of small renal calculi in general, but particularly in overweight patients. While SWL machines with shock frequencies up to 180/minute are now available, thus shortening the duration of each treatment considerably, it would appear that lower frequencies are associated with improved stone fragmentation rates.[26]

References

1. Best S, Ercole B, Lee C et al. Minimally invasive therapy for renal cell carcinoma: is there a new community standard? *Urology* 2004;64:22–5.

2. Permpongkosol S, Chan DY, Link RE et al. Long-term survival analysis after laparoscopic radical nephrectomy. *J Urol* 2005;174:1222–5.

3. Kato M, Suzuki T, Suzuki Y et al. Natural history of small renal cell carcinoma: evaluation of growth rate, histological grade, cell proliferation and apoptosis. *J Urol* 2004;172: 863–6.

4. Gill IS, Colombo JR Jr, Frank I et al. Laparoscopic partial nephrectomy for hilar tumors. *J Urol* 2005;174:850–3.

5. Finelli A, Gill IS, Desai MM et al. Laparoscopic heminephrectomy for tumor. *Urology* 2005;65:473–8.

6. Laven BA, Orvieo MA, Chuang MS et al. Renal tolerance to prolonged warm ischemia time in a laparoscopic versus open surgery porcine model. *J Urol* 2004;172:2471–4.

7. Desai MM, Gill IS, Ramani AP et al. The impact of warm ischemia on renal function after laparoscopic partial nephrectomy. *BJU Int* 2005;95:377–83.

8. Gill IS, Remer EM, Hasan WM et al. Renal cryoablation: outcome at 3 years. *J Urol* 2005;173:1903–7.

9. Shingleton WB, Siskron T, D'Agostino H. Percutaneous renal cryoablation with computerized tomography guidance. *J Endourol* 2005;19:A108.

10. Silverman SG, Tuncali K, van Sonnenberg E et al. Renal tumors: MR imaging-guided percutaneous cryotherapy – initial experience in 23 patients. *Radiology* 2005;236:716–24.

11. Johnson DB, Solomon SB, Su LM et al. Defining complications of cryoablation and radio frequency ablation of small renal tumors: a multi-institutional review. *J Urol* 2004;172:874–7.

12. Matsumoto ED, Johnson DB, Ogan K et al. Short-term efficacy of temperature-based radiofrequency ablation of small renal tumors. *Urology* 2005;65:877–81.

13. Ahlering TE, Woo D, Eichel L et al. Robot-assisted versus open radical prostatectomy: a comparison of one surgeon's outcomes. *Urology* 2004;63:819–22.

14. Lotan Y, Caddedu JA, Gettman MT. The new economics of radical prostatectomy: cost comparison of open, laparoscopic and robot assisted prostatectomy. *J Urol* 2004;172:1431–5.

15. Menon M, Kaul S, Bhandari A et al. Potency following robotic radical prostatectomy: a questionnaire based analysis of outcomes after conventional nerve sparing and prostatic fascia sparing techniques. *J Urol* 2005;174:2291–6.

16. Ukimura O, Gill IS, Desai MM et al. Real-time transrectal ultrasonography during laparoscopic radical prostatectomy. *J Urol* 2004;172:112–18.

17. Gill IS, Ukimura O, Rubinstein M et al. Lateral pedicle control during laparoscopic radical prostatectomy: refined technique. *Urology* 2005;65: 23–7.

18. Ahlering TE, Eichel L, Chou D, Skarecky DW. Feasibility study for robotic radical prostatectomy cautery-free neurovascular bundle preservation. *Urology* 2005;65:994–7.

19. Prepelica KL, Okeke Z, Murphy A, Katz AE. Cryosurgical ablation of the prostate: high risk patient outcomes. *Cancer* 2005;103:1625–30.

20. Uchida T, Ohkusa H, Nagata Y et al. Treatment of localized prostate cancer using high-intensity focused ultrasound. *BJU Int* 2006;97:56–61.

21. Cathalineau X, Arroyo C, Rozet F et al. Laparoscopic assisted radical cystectomy: the Montsouris experience after 84 cases. *Eur Urol* 2005;47:780–4.

22. Preminger GM, Assimos DG, Lingeman JE et al.; AUA Nephrolithiasis Guideline Panel. Chapter 1: AUA guideline on management of staghorn calculi: diagnosis and treatment recommendations. *J Urol* 2005; 173:1991–2000.

23. Wickham JEA, Miller RA, Kellett MJ, Payne SR. Percutaneous nephrolithotomy: one stage or two? *Br J Urol* 1984;56:582–5.

24. Shah HN, Kausik VB, Hegde SS et al. Safety and efficacy of bilateral simultaneous tubeless percutaneous nephrolithotomy. *Urology* 2005;66:500–4.

25. Taylor EN, Stampfer MJ, Curhan GC. Obesity, weight gain, and the risk of kidney stones. *JAMA* 2005;293:455–62.

26. Pace KT, Ghiculete D, Harju M, Honey RJ. Shock wave lithotripsy at 60 or 120 shocks: a randomized, double-blind trial. *J Urol* 2005; 174:595–9.

Mathialagan Murugesan Dip(Urol) FRCS and
Senthil Nathan FRCS(Edin) FEBU FRCS(Urol) MPhil(Urol)

Department of Urology, Whittington Hospital, London, UK

Continuing its historic tradition, urology is again at the forefront of rapid development and implementation of new technologies. These are having a major impact on both diagnosis and management. This chapter describes new techniques that have been implemented recently and some that are in development. It is by no means comprehensive and readers are advised to refer to the references listed. Approvals granted by licensing authorities like the US Food and Drug Administration (FDA) and the European Union (EU) are mentioned.

Diagnostics

New diagnostic methods for urologic malignancies, particularly prostate cancer, are always being researched. Most have not reached clinical usage, but some major advances have occurred in the last 2 years.

uPM3™ test for prostate cancer. This test for a genetic marker in urine samples was developed by Bostwick Laboratories (Richmond, VA, USA).[1] The uPM3 test is based on $DD3^{PCA3}$, a gene that is expressed profusely by prostate cancer tissue (on average at a level 34 times higher than in benign prostate tissue). No other human tissue has been shown to express $DD3^{PCA3}$. The test has a sensitivity of 67% and a specificity of 89% for predicting prostate cancer.

The test is performed on the initial 10 mL urine obtained after a prostate massage. It uses the isothermic nucleic-acid-based amplification method. Prostate-specific antigen (PSA) mRNA and PCA3 RNA, which are selectively expressed in prostate cancer, are detected simultaneously using real-time spectrofluorometry. The test is particularly useful when a negative biopsy is reported in patients for whom there is a strong suspicion of prostate cancer. The uPM3 test is now available for clinical use.

U-M test for prostate cancer. Researchers from the University of Michigan have recently published results of a new blood test for the diagnosis of prostate cancer.[2] Patients with cancer produce autoantibodies against oncoproteins. The researchers scanned a library of 2300 autoantibodies, 186 of which reacted with blood serum from men with prostate cancer. Of these 186 autoantibodies, 22 were found to react consistently with prostate cancer oncoproteins in significant proportions. The test has a sensitivity of 88% and specificity of 82%. Results of a larger clinical trial are awaited and should be available soon. The U-M test is not yet available for clinical use.

Urinary telomerase activity for bladder cancer. Urinary telomerase activity, determined by a telemetric repeat amplification protocol (TRAP) assay, has been recently found to be a highly sensitive and specific urinary marker for bladder cancer, including grade 1 tumors. In a prospective study, Sanchini and colleagues measured telomerase levels in voided urine specimens from 84 healthy men and 134 men with bladder cancer.[3] Sensitivity was 93%, 87% and 89% for grade 1, 2 and 3 tumors, respectively (Table 1). In contrast, cytology was sensitive in 46.6%. The test is about to become commercially available and may play a significant role in the screening and follow-up of bladder cancer.

Imaging
Major advances have been made in this field, particularly in relation to diagnosis and planning treatment for urologic malignancies.

Combination of magnetic resonance imaging (MRI) and magnetic resonance spectroscopic imaging (MRSI) in prostate cancer staging. MRSI is a technique based on MRI that delineates tissues

TABLE 1

Median sensitivity (%) of urinary telomerase activity measurement per grade of urinary markers for transitional cell carcinoma[4]

Grade	BTA	BTA stat	NMP22	Telomerase	Cytology
1	31	45	56	93	17
2	43	60	77	87	34
3	50	75	81	89	58

BTA, bladder tumor antigen; NMP, nuclear matrix protein.

biologically. In prostate cancer, the cellular content of choline, creatine and citrate are estimated. In 85 men with prostate cancer, MRSI before radical prostatectomy[5] detected significantly higher choline levels and significantly lower citrate levels in cancerous than in benign tissue. MRI on its own predicts positive margins with a sensitivity of 79%. By combining MRI and MRSI, the sensitivity increases to 91%, with a significant impact on treatment choice.

Restitu Restore three-dimensional imaging system. Failure of accurate targeting is known to be a major cause of radiotherapy failure. Targeting fails because of non-reproducible patient positioning on the X-ray table, variation in prostate dimensions and minor movements of the prostate within the pelvis.

Resonant Medical (Montreal, Canada) has developed a three-dimensional imaging system that merges images from computed tomography (CT) and transrectal ultrasound. Three-dimensional images are calibrated during planning and are accurately reproduced during delivery of radiation. As it is a dynamic process for each treatment, variables such as patient position on the table and prostate size are taken into account. It is envisaged that this imaging will allow radiotherapy to be more accurate, and thus to increase its efficacy and reduce its toxicity.

Target scan system for prostate biopsy and treatment is an innovative development in which the ultrasound probe remains stationary and the transducers within the housing move in different planes to present a three-dimensional image of the prostate, eliminating the need to physically move the probe during the procedure and preventing displacement of the gland. It allows better targeting and placement of radioactive seeds for brachytherapy and needles for cryotherapy. Envisioneering Medical Technologies (St Louis, MO, USA) has received FDA approval to market the system.

Treatment

There is no long-term or class 1 evidence for the treatment modalities described below, despite their rapid diffusion.

Transurethral microwave thermotherapy (TUMT). CoreTherm (ProstaLund, Lund, Sweden) is a third-generation transurethral microwave treatment useful in benign prostatic hyperplasia (BPH).[6] A catheter that contains a microwave antenna and an intraprostatic probe generates temperatures of 45–50°C, causing coagulative necrosis of the prostate. Three temperature sensors are present in the catheter to allow for variable prostate size. This outpatient procedure can be performed under local anesthesia. The results of TUMT are comparable to those with transurethral resection of the prostate (TURP) but morbidity is lower. Urinary retention, dysuria, urethral discharge and bleeding are common side effects. A urinary catheter is placed after treatment and is removed after a week.

Transurethral microwave dilatation (TUMD) is a new technique to treat BPH. This dual-action thermodilatation technology simultaneously heats the prostate and dilates the urethra. The procedure is performed as day surgery under local anesthesia and does not require catheterization. Results of preliminary trials are awaited.

Photoselective vaporization of the prostate (PVP). KTP-YAG (potassium titanyl phosphate–yttrium aluminum garnet) laser

105

vaporization of the prostate is similar to electrovaporization. The green light is selectively absorbed by the heme in red blood cells, vaporizing tissue at more than 100°C. The delivery mechanism is through a semi-rigid rod, allowing pinpoint targeting using a cystoscope. The KTP-YAG laser uses a peak power of 280 W with short pulse frequency. This allows high-density energy to be deposited in a shallow layer of tissue, with an optical penetration of approximately 0.8 mm, producing a coagulation zone of 1–2 mm so that the targeted superficial tissue can reach the vaporization threshold of greater than 100°C. The procedure results in a wide open cavity with shreds of necrotized tissue lining the wall; these are voided over a period of 4 weeks. The procedure can be performed as a day case or extended day case under regional or general anesthesia. Many patients do not require a catheter, and those who do are typically catheterized for less than 24 hours. Postoperative dysuria and secondary hemorrhage are frequent early complications. Preliminary results are encouraging, and it will be interesting to see the long-term outcomes.

HoLAP (holmium laser ablation of the prostate) and HoLEP (holmium laser enucleation of the prostate). The holmium:YAG laser has widespread urologic applications, particularly in the treatment of urolithiasis. The holmium laser has an absorption depth of 0.5 mm or less, and hemostasis with holmium is remarkably good. Its localized coagulation effect seals the tissue and provides hemostasis superior to that achieved with electrocautery instruments, without producing the thermal injury associated with Nd:YAG or KTP lasers. The holmium coagulation effect minimizes fluid absorption more effectively than electrocautery. The ablating and hemostasis features of holmium make it an excellent energy choice for treatment of BPH; HoLAP and HoLEP are two options that can be used to treat BPH effectively.[7]

Use of the holmium:YAG laser in the treatment of BPH has changed significantly over the last 5 years. As techniques have been refined and equipment improved, treatment has progressed from simple vaporization to complete enucleation. HoLEP with mechanical morcellation represents the latest refinement of the technique.

Gyrus Plasmasect loop bipolar TURP. Gyrus Group (London, UK) has introduced a new resection loop that uses bipolar current rather than the traditional monopolar TURP loops. A preliminary study comparing bipolar and monopolar resection showed no significant differences in terms of efficacy.[8] However, blood loss was smaller and postoperative catheterization time and hospital stay were shorter in the bipolar current group. Importantly, prostate chips are available for histology.

Cryoablation of the prostate. New third-generation cryotherapy systems (Figure 1) have been developed with controlled ice-ball formation and warming techniques. SeedNet™ (Galil Medical, Woburn, MA, USA), and Cryocare® (Endocare, Irvine, CA, USA) are similar mechanisms that are safe and effective treatments for prostate cancer.[9] Using transrectal ultrasound, 18F hollow needles are positioned in the prostate. Two cycles of rapid freezing to below

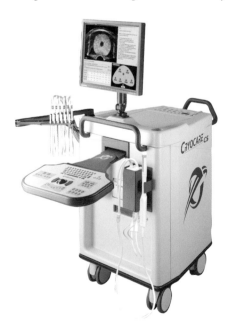

Figure 1 Cryotherapy for prostate cancer: the Cryocare system. Image courtesy of Endocare.

–40°C and slow thawing effectively destroy prostate tissue. The process is constantly monitored with thermosensors and transrectal ultrasound and is fine-tuned as necessary. It is a choice for curative treatment in localized prostate cancer (T1, T2 and T3a) and for patients in whom radiotherapy or brachytherapy has failed.[10]

High-intensity focused ultrasound (HIFU). HIFU has been used in the management of prostatic disease for nearly 2 decades, mainly for BPH. HIFU is a non-invasive acoustic ablation technique that uses intersecting, tightly focused ultrasound waves to raise the temperature of the target tissues to more than 80°C. Ultrasound energy is non-ionizing and does not affect tissues surrounding the target zone, in contrast to radiation therapies. Its use in localized prostate cancer has recently been reported in *Nature*.[11] Results from four centers were reviewed from 1997 to February 2005. The success rate, as evidenced by negative biopsies after 1 year, was 93.4% for primary and salvage patients.

Photodynamic therapy (PDT) for men with untreated localized prostate cancer. Cancer Research UK started recruiting patients with localized prostate cancer for PDT from 2004. PDT uses photosensitizing molecules that, when treated with electromagnetic radiation of certain wavelengths, transfer the absorbed energy to the neighboring molecules. The therapeutic effect is augmented when the tumor cells accumulate photosensitizing molecules that are either produced within the body (internal photosensitizers) or introduced from without (external photosensitizers). Irradiation at the correct wavelength induces a photochemical reaction that results in necrosis or modification of malignant cells so that they can be recognized by the immune system. Researchers are using a new photosensitizing drug, WSTO9, for which results are awaited in 2007.

Erectile dysfunction and infertility
Intra-vas device. Shepherd Medical (Vancouver, Canada) has introduced a flexible, hollow, silicone plug that can be inserted into the vas deferens with a special needle, in order to block sperm

transport. The device is inserted under local anesthesia after isolation of the vas deferens and can be removed, re-establishing sperm flow, if the patient desires. FDA approval is awaited.

Gradi flow: the sperm separator. Scientists at the University of Newcastle, New South Wales, Australia, have developed a device to separate healthy sperm from damaged ones, for use in assisted conception. It works on the principle that the sperm with the most negatively charged membranes are likely to have the least DNA damage. The device consists of two chambers separated by a filter. The sperm are injected into the first chamber and a voltage is applied across the filter to move negatively charged, undamaged sperm to the second chamber.

The 'Viagra' condom. Future Medical, a British company, has developed the CSD500 condom, which incorporates an erectogenic compound (glyceryl trinitrate). The idea is to maintain erection following ejaculation to prevent condom slippage. It will also prevent semen spillage resulting from detumescence. It is believed that this will encourage condom use and safe sex. EU marketing authorization is awaited.

Eros therapy. Female sexual dysfunction is now a well-established clinical entity. The Eros clitoral therapy device (UroMetrics, St Paul, MN, USA) mimics the male vacuum devices for erectile dysfunction. A small soft cup is placed over the clitoris and a low vacuum applied. It increases clitoral blood flow, resulting in improved sexual response and attainment of climax. The device has received FDA approval and is available on prescription only.

Incontinence

Urgent neuromodulation for incontinence. The FDA has approved sale of a new device to prevent incontinence – the Urgent® PC Neuromodulation System (Figure 2) from Uroplasty (Minneapolis, MN, USA). A percutaneous needle is inserted 5 cm cephalad to the medial malleolus and connected to a stimulator, and an electrical

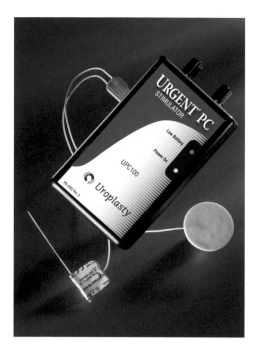

Figure 2 The Urgent® PC Neuromodulation System. (Image courtesy of Uroplasty.)

current is applied. The amplitude is slowly increased until the patient's hallux starts to flex, indicating proximity to the tibial nerve. Electrical impulses travel retrograde via the tibial and sacral nerves to the sacral segments. From here, impulses regulate bladder and pelvic floor function. The patient is treated weekly for 30 minutes. Significant reductions in frequency and urgency have been reported after approximately 12 weeks.[12]

This technique can also be used to treat pelvic pain syndromes.

Intravesical botulinum toxin in overactive bladder. Intravesical injection of botulinum toxin has been tried for many overactive bladder syndromes, with varied responses. There are seven botulinum toxins (A–G), all of which are powerful neurotoxins that block the release of acetylcholine at the neuromuscular junction. In a randomized placebo-controlled study on botulinum toxin type A, Schurch and colleagues reported significant efficacy in the treatment of urinary incontinence caused by detrusor hyperreflexia in people with spinal-cord injury.[13] Compared with the placebo group, patients receiving a single injection of botulinum toxin type A, 200 U or 300 U, into the detrusor muscle experienced a reduction in episodes of incontinence, improved bladder function and improved quality of life over a 6-month period, with no significant adverse effects.

The effects of botulinum toxin B on refractory detrusor overactivity were recently tested in a randomized, double-blind, placebo-controlled, crossover trial. There were statistically significant improvements in voided volume, urinary frequency and episodes of incontinence in the active treatment compared with the placebo groups.[14]

Botulinum toxin A has also been used in interstitial cystitis, non-bacterial prostatitis and BPH.

Intraurethral device for voiding dysfunction in women. The Inflow Catheter (SRS Medical, Billerica, MA, USA) is a new intraurethral device composed of a short silicone catheter containing an internal valve.[15] It has an external remote control that activates a pump in the device to facilitate voiding. The device is fixed in position by flexible silicone fins at the bladder neck and by a flexible flange at the external meatus. In the core of the valve and pump mechanism is a small magnet, which is energized remotely by a flow activator. To operate the mechanism, the activator is held at the pubic area near the urethral opening and activated. The valve opens and the miniature rotor spins at a speed of 10 000 rpm. The pump draws urine from the bladder and the patient voids with an average urine flow of 10–12 mL per second. The In-Flow Catheter is available in different sizes for an effective fit.

The LifePort® kidney transporter

This is a new hypothermic organ perfuser and transporter for cadaveric kidneys (Figure 3), developed by Organ Recovery Systems (Chicago, IL, USA). The device perfuses the kidney from the time of retrieval to transplantation. It comprises simplified connections with customized, disposable cannulas and tube sets. It ensures stability

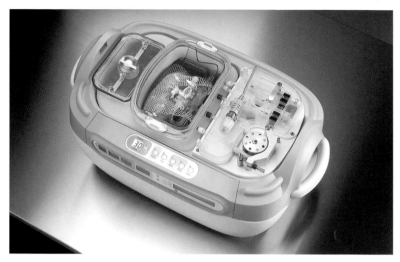

Figure 3 The LifePort® kidney transporter. (Image courtesy of Organ Recovery Systems.)

and protection during transit and also monitors and displays vital organ function in real time.

Robotics and telesurgery

This chapter would be incomplete without mention of robotics and telesurgery. Surgical robots are of active and passive types. The former work independently after programming, while the latter help the surgeon to target tissues accurately. Surgical robots were initially trialed in neurosurgery, orthopedics and urology. In fact, the Probot, a urologic robot, was the first robot in the world to actively remove pieces of tissue from the human body, in this instance the prostate. Since then, passive robots that assist percutaneous renal access, transperineal prostate biopsy and radioactive seed delivery into the prostate have been developed.[16]

Telesurgery comprises passive target guidance and master–slave systems. The best developed master–slave systems that are not true robots are the Zeus and da Vinci® systems (Computer Motion, Goleta, CA, USA, and Intuitive Surgical, Sunnyvale, CA, USA, respectively). The da Vinci robot (Figure 4) is used in many centers to perform laparoscopic nephrectomy, cystectomy and radical

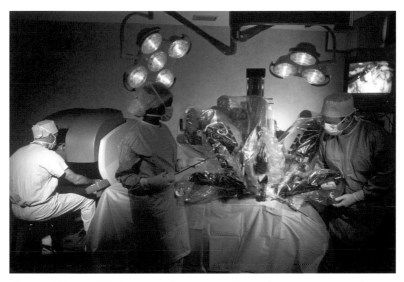

Figure 4 The da Vinci master–slave system in use (image courtesy of Intuitive Surgical).

prostatectomy. It has the unique qualities of six degrees of movement, which is better than the human hand, and tremor filtration.

Robotic assistance has proved to be of great assistance in performing the procedures listed above. With the addition of three-dimensional views, the da Vinci has nullified the need for expert spatial orientation in laparoscopic surgery. Tactile instruments are being developed for a better feel of the tissues.[17,18]

Telesurgery integrates multimedia, telecommunications and robotic technologies to provide surgical care at a distance. Through telesurgical mentoring, surgeons with basic laparoscopic skills could receive training in an advanced technique from a world expert without the need to travel. The first telesurgical urologic procedure was carried out between Baltimore and Rome in 1998, using a passive surgical robot PAKY (percutaneous access to the kidney).[19] Substantial progress has since been made in developing telesurgical systems that can be modified for complex robotic telesurgery.

Highlights in recent technological advances in urology 2005–06

WHAT'S IN?

- uPM3 genetic marker for prostate cancer
- NMP22 urinary marker for bladder transitional cell carcinoma
- Green-light laser photoselective vaporization of the prostate
- Magnetic resonance imaging scan of the pelvis for prostate cancer staging
- Gyrus plasmasect bipolar loop transurethral resection of the prostate
- Cryotherapy for localized cancer of the prostate

WHAT'S OUT?

- Prostate-specific antigen density measurement
- Bladder tumor antigen (BTA) and BTA stat markers for bladder transitional cell carcinoma
- Computed tomography staging for prostate cancer
- Gyrus electrovaporization of the prostate

References

1. Fradet Y, Saad F, Aprikian A et al. uPM3, a new molecular urine test for the detection of prostate cancer. *Urology* 2004;64:311–15.

2. Finn OJ. Immune response as a biomarker for cancer detection and a lot more. *N Engl J Med* 2005;353:1288–90.

3. Sanchini MA, Gunelli R, Nanni O et al. Relevance of urine telomerase in the diagnosis of bladder cancer. *JAMA* 2005;294:2052–6.

4. van Rhijn BW, van der Poel HG, van der Kwast TH. Urine markers for bladder cancer surveillance: a systematic review. *Eur Urol* 2005;47:736–48.

5. Wood P, Kurhanewicz J, Vigneron D et al. The role of combined MRI and MRSI in treating prostate cancer. *PCRI Insights* 2000;3.2(August). www.prostate-cancer.org/education/staging/UCSF_CombinedMRI_MRSI.html

6. CoreTherm for BPH ablation. *MedGadget, Internet Journal of Emerging Medical Technologies* 2005; May 25. www.medgadget.com/archives/2005/05/coretherm_for_b.html

7. Moody JA, Lingeman JE. Holmium laser enucleation for prostate adenoma greater than 100 gm: comparison to open prostatectomy. *J Urol* 2001;165: 459–62.

8. Yang S, Lin WC, Chang HK et al. Gyrus Plasmasect: is it better than monopolar transurethral resection of prostate? *Urol Int* 2004;73:258–61.

9. Bahn DK, Lee F, Badalament R et al. Targeted cryoablation of the prostate: 7-year outcomes in the primary treatment of prostate cancer: *Urology* 2002 60(2 suppl 1):3–11.

10. Shabbir M, Dovey Z, Ghei M et al. Salvage cryosurgery for recurrent localized prostate cancer. *Proceedings of the British Prostate Group Spring Meeting,* 11 April 2005. www.britishprostategroup.co.uk/abstracts.htm.

11. Chaussy C, Thüroff S, Rebillard X, Gelet A. Technology Insight: high-intensity focused ultrasound for urologic cancers. *Nat Clin Pract Urol* 2005;2:191–8.

12. Congregado Ruiz B, Pena Outeirino XM, Campoy Martinez P et al. Peripheral afferent nerve stimulation for treatment of lower urinary tract irritative symptoms. *Eur Urol* 2004;45:65–9.

13. Schurch B, de Seze M, Denys P et al. Botox Detrusor Hyperreflexia Study Team. Botulinum toxin type A is a safe and effective treatment for neurogenic urinary incontinence: results of a single treatment, randomized, placebo controlled 6-month study. *J Urol* 2005;174: 196–200.

14. Ghei M, Maraj BA, Miller R et al. Effects of botulinum toxin B on refractory detrusor overactivity: a randomized, double-blind, placebo controlled, crossover trial. *J Urol* 2005;174:1873–7.

15. Madjar S, Sabo E, Halachmi S et al. A remote controlled intraurethral insert for artificial voiding: a new concept for treating women with voiding dysfunction. *J Urol* 1999;161:895–8.

16. Nathan S, Wickham JEA. Robotic transurethral electrovaporisation of the prostate. *Minim Invasive Ther Allied Technol* 1995;5:292–6.

17. Hemal AK, Menon M. Laparoscopy, robot, telesurgery and urology: future perspective. *J Postgrad Med* 2002;48:39–41.

18. Tewari A, Srivasatava A, Menon M; members of the VIP Team. A prospective comparison of radical retropubic and robot-assisted prostatectomy: experience in one institution. *BJU Int* 2003;92:205–10.

19. Cadeseddu JA, Stoianovici D, Chen RN et al. Stereotactic mechanical percutaneous renal access. *J Endourol* 1998;12:121–5.